MINDS, BRAINS, AND LEARNING

Minds, Brains, and Learning

Understanding the Psychological and Educational Relevance of Neuroscientific Research

James P. Byrnes

THE GUILFORD PRESS
New York London

© 2001 The Guilford Press
A Division of Guilford Publications, Inc.
72 Spring Street, New York, NY 10012
www.guilford.com

Printed in the United States of America

This book is printed on acid-free paper.

Last digit is print number: 9 8 7 6 5 4 3 2

Library of Congress Cataloging-in-Publication Data

Byrnes, James P.
    Minds, brains, and learning: understanding the psychological and
  educational relevance of neuroscientific research / James P. Byrnes.
      p. cm.
  Includes bibliographical references and index.
  ISBN 1-57230-651-3 (hardcover)—ISBN 1-57230-652-1 (pbk.)
  1. Cognitive neuroscience. 2. Neuropsychology. 3. Learning,
  Psychology of. I. Title.

QP360.5 .B97 2001
612.8′2—dc21   00-067750

To Clare M. Byrnes, *who has fostered
the development of my mind, brain,
and soul for so many years*

About the Author

James P. Byrnes, PhD, is a Professor of Human Development in the College of Education at the University of Maryland, College Park, where he is affiliated with the Neuroscience and Cognitive Science program. He has published research in the areas of mathematics learning, decision making, language, deductive reasoning, gender differences in cognition, and ethnic differences in school achievement. He is former vice president of the Jean Piaget Society and serves on the editorial boards of a number of journals, including the *Journal of Educational Psychology, Child Development, American Educational Research Journal,* and the *Journal of Cognition and Development.*

Preface

This book began as a challenge that I posed to myself back in the fall of 1994. At that time, I was a staunch advocate of the position that there is nothing to be gained from a consideration of brain research. I am a psychologist, after all, not a biologist. And yet I was worried that I was engaging in the same sort of closed-minded thinking that has stifled scientific progress so many times over the years. In addition, some of my closest and most respected colleagues were embracing brain research with vigor. To make sure that I was not missing something important, I decided to teach a graduate course on brain research. My goal was to become familiar enough with the literature to see right through it. Much to my surprise, I ended up convincing myself that brain research could be highly relevant to the fields of education and psychology if this research is viewed in a particular light. I summarized what I learned in this process in a paper that I wrote with my colleague Nathan Fox (Byrnes & Fox, 1998). Chris Jennison at The Guilford Press read the paper and thought that it might make an excellent book if expanded considerably. The present book represents the expanded version of the original paper.

The intended audience includes three kinds of people: (1) psychologists who are highly skeptical of the relevance of brain research (or perhaps just on the fence), (2) teachers and others in the field of education who are currently being bombarded with information about the brain in teacher-oriented publications and professional development seminars, and (3) anyone else who wants to know more about the brain but is intimidated by the considerable size and complexity of the neuroscientific literature. It is my hope that my skeptical colleagues in psychology will lose some of their skepticism after reading this book. In addition, I will accomplish something important if educators who read this book learn enough to tell the difference between plausible applications of brain research and unfounded speculations. Finally, I hope that those who are merely curious about the brain will learn a great deal and be motivated to learn more. Although practicing neuroscientists are probably already familiar with much of the content of this book, I think they too could benefit from seeing how someone who is not steeped in the intellectual tradition of neuroscience views their work.

I would like to express my gratitude to the following groups of individuals. The first group includes the graduate students who participated in my course on the brain in the fall of 1994: Donetta Cochran, Vic Emerson, Mary Ann Krehbiel, Cedric Lynch, Mary Jo Primosch, Todd Riniolo, Susan Robertson, Mark Stout, Carolyn Veiga, and Maryanne Reynolds. In many ways, their enthusiasm and comments helped me to see the wisdom of learning from brain research. The second group includes colleagues who read and commented on the original Byrnes and Fox (1998) paper or on the first draft of this book: Lou Schmidt, Todd Riniolo, Mike Pressley, Keith Stanovich, Ginger Berninger, David Corina, Dave Bjorklund, Rhonda Douglas Brown, David Geary, Rich Mayer, Michael O'Boyle, Harwant Gill, Dale Schunk, Merlin Wittrock, Steve Benton, and Michael S. Meloth. I modified my original position to address many of their excellent points, but the views expressed here are my own. Next I want to thank Nathan Fox, my coauthor on the original paper, for his expert advice and for inviting me to interact with colleagues in his lab. In addition, I am grateful to Chris Jennison at The Guilford Press for encouraging me to write this book in the first place and for his excellent shepherding of the project from beginning to end. Finally, I want to thank my wife, Barbara Wasik, and children, Julia and Tommy, for supporting me with their love and patience while I wrote this book.

Contents

CHAPTER 1

Introduction

For many centuries, scholars from a variety of disciplines have been interested in the neural basis of thinking and learning. During the Renaissance, for example, philosophers such as René Descartes wondered how a material thing (the brain) could produce, or make contact with, an immaterial thing (the mind). Somewhat later, physicians and physiologists became intrigued by the curious deficits that sometimes occur when people experience brain injuries (Posner & Raichle, 1994). With the advent of the field of psychology in the late 1800s, a variety of new questions arose regarding the links between the brain and the mind. Even so, relatively few psychologists explored these links in a systematic way because of the common perception that brain functioning was not a matter of concern to psychologists. In many ways, this sense of the irrelevance of brain research still pervades much of psychology. However, a growing number of psychologists have apparently begun to change their opinion in recent years (Byrnes & Fox, 1998). For example, whereas only a handful of articles on cognition in the 1980s took a neuroscientific slant, a large number of cognition articles published in the 1990s focused on the neural basis of cognition and learning.

What precipitated this apparent change in perspective? Several historical trends can be identified. The first was the emergence of the field of *cognitive science* in the late 1980s. From its inception, the goal of cognitive science has been to bring together scholars from a variety of disciplines who have a mutual interest in the study of intelligence. Two key disciplines that were brought together in this collaborative enterprise were cognitive psychology and neuroscience (Posner & Raichle, 1994). The second precipitating event was the rise of the *connectionist approach* to cognition. A central premise of connectionism is that theoretical models of cognition should be based on current knowledge of brain functioning (Rumelhart, 1989). The third precipitating event was the development and increased availability of brain-imaging techniques (e.g., *positron emission tomography* and *functional magnetic resonance imaging*) that provide glimpses of brain activity as an individual engages in cognitive and emotional processing (Posner & Raichle, 1994). The fourth precipitating event was the passage of congressional resolutions that designated the 1990s as "the decade of the brain" (Wolfe & Brandt, 1998). Among other things, these resolutions prompted certain federal agencies to fund more neuroscientific endeavors.

Collectively, these four trends have created an atmosphere of increased (though certainly not universal) acceptance of the idea that neuroscientific research could provide the answers to important questions about learning and cognition. But I must underscore my use of the term "could" here. Most scholars believe that the available neuroscientific evidence is provocative and interesting, but far from conclusive. Regrettably, this fact has not stopped some authors and journalists from mischaracterizing and overinterpreting what has been found (Bruer, 1997; Byrnes & Fox, 1998). One of my goals in this book is to help the reader discriminate between the kinds of inferences that can be currently supported by neuroscientific evidence, and the kinds of inferences that cannot be so supported. In each chapter, I will critically analyze the results of certain studies using questions such as: (1) Are the findings credible and valid? and (2) Are the findings consistent across studies? By repeatedly asking such questions, the reader will learn how to avoid some of the unwarranted inferences that have appeared in the popular press in recent years. In Chapter 8, I describe and critique specific examples of these inferences using information in this book.

My goal in the present chapter is to provide an interpretive context for the chapters that follow. In the next section, I shall examine some of the arguments that have been advanced over the years regarding the irrelevance of neuroscientific evidence for psychological questions. Then, I will define and illustrate some essential neuroscientific terms (including labels of important brain structures and regions). Next, I will describe and critique the unique methodologies used by neuroscientists. Finally, I will briefly preview the content of the remaining chapters. Readers who are already familiar with the matters covered in the first three sections can skip to the final section.

ARGUMENTS FOR AND AGAINST
THE RELEVANCE OF BRAIN RESEARCH

Although the number of psychologists and educators who hold positive attitudes regarding brain research has grown in recent years, the majority of individuals in these fields still see little value in this research for their own work or for the training of students. In departments of psychology or human development, for example, it is sometimes hard to find support for the idea that all students need to take courses on the physiological basis of psychological phenomena. The usual argument against offering such courses is that psychologists and educators can get along quite well without knowing anything at all about the brain. In addition to their own personal experience in this regard, faculty members who are unfamiliar with brain research can turn to influential papers written by prominent individuals to bolster their case. Before reviewing the neuroscientific evidence, then, it would seem that the first order of business is to consider the merits of some of the arguments against the relevance of brain research.

Argument 1: The Computer Analog

Several variants of the computer analogy have appeared over the years. The basic premise is that the human brain is analogous to the hardware of a computer. The mind, in contrast, is analogous to the software of a computer. As Neisser (1967, p. 6) wrote,

> The task of a psychologist trying to understand human cognition is analogous to that of a man trying to discover how a computer has been programmed. In particular, if the program seems to store and reuse information, he would like to know by what "routines" or "procedures" this is done. Given this purpose, he will not care much whether his particular computer stores information in magnetic codes or in thin films; he wants to understand the program, not the "hardware." . . . He wants to understand its utilization, not its incarnation.

In a similar way, Marr (1982) suggested that there are three levels at which some psychological process could be characterized by a theorist: the computational level, the algorithmic level, and the implementation level. The *computational* level describes the primary task to be performed by some system or individual (e.g., find the area under a curve). The *algorithmic* level describes the steps taken by a particular individual when that individual performs the task in question (e.g., uses calculus vs. measures the area with a ruler). The *implementation* level describes the mechanisms by which the algorithm is carried out in some physical system (e.g., a brain or a computer). Marr argued that when researchers are trying to create a computer simulation of some cognitive process (e.g., vision), they can temporarily ignore implementation issues when they are working on issues at the computational and algorithmic levels. In other words, they need not worry about such things as whether the program will run on a Macintosh or an IBM when they are considering what the task will be and what algorithm will be used to accomplish the task. Many scholars have used Marr's account to argue that psychologists normally operate at the computational and algorithmic levels when they construct theories of mental events. As such, they, too, do not have to be concerned about implementation issues (i.e., how the brain manages to carry out some cognitive process).

The computer analogy is part of a larger and very influential paradigm known as the *computational theory of mind* (Block, 1990; Pylyshyn, 1989). The basic claim of the computational theory is that "the mind is the program of the brain and that the mechanisms of the mind involve the same sorts of computations over representations that occur in computers" (Block, 1990, p. 247). For my present purposes, the details of this claim are less important than the ultimate realization that

> the computer model of the mind is profoundly *unbiological*. We are beings who have a useful and interesting biological level of description, but the computer model aims for a level of description of the mind that abstracts away from the biological realizations of cognitive structures. . . . Of course, this is not to say that the computer model is in any way incompatible with a biological approach. Indeed, cooperation between the biological and computational approaches is vital to *discovering* the program of the brain. . . . Nonetheless, the computer model of mind has a built-in antibiological bias in the following sense. If the computer model is right, we should be able to create intelligent systems in our image. . . . It is an open empirical question whether or not the computer model of mind is correct. Only if it is *not* correct could it be said that psychology, the science of mind, is a biological science. (Block, 1990, p. 261)

In effect, then, psychologists and educators could easily appeal to the still-dominant computational theory of mind to defend their claim that neuroscientific questions are somewhat irrelevant. For example, an educator could say, "I am only interested in the strategies children use to solve math problems [i.e., the algorithmic level]. I am not interested in the biological mechanisms responsible for their brains' ability to envision and carry out these strategies [i.e., the implementation level]. How would knowing the latter make me a better teacher?"

This is obviously a good question and one that is based on a compelling line of argumentation (that I have only touched on here). The key to finding flaws in this line of argumentation is to consider the ways in which the computer analogy of mind is either misleading or incorrect.

Rumelhart (1989, p. 134) adopts the former approach and suggests that Marr's three-levels account is

> true for computers because they are essentially the same. Whether we make them out of vacuum tubes or transistors, and whether we use an IBM or an Apple computer, we are using computers of the same general design. When we look at an essentially different architecture [e.g., the brain], we see that the architecture makes a great deal of difference. It is the architecture which determines which kinds of algorithms are most easily carried out on the machine in question. It is the architecture of the machine that determines the essential nature of the program itself. It is thus reasonable that we should begin by asking what we know about the architecture of the brain and how it might shape the algorithms underlying biological intelligence and human mental life.

To extend Rumelhart's argument somewhat, consider the following. Would an aviation expert ignore the object that is flying when he or she is providing a theoretical account of this object's flight (Iran-Nejad, Hidi, & Wittrock, 1992)? A little reflection shows that the answer is clearly no. An explanation of how a bird manages to fly would differ in important respects from an explanation of how an airplane flies. Similarly, would a physicist ignore the molecular structure of particular magnets when he or she is explaining the functioning of magnets? Again, the answer would be no. Some objects are only magnetic when electricity is running through them, others can be permanently magnetized, while still others can only be temporarily magnetized. Hence, the thing that is flying or attracting metal is clearly important. If we failed to think about the object involved, we would never really develop a useful or accurate theory of flight or of magnetism. In the same way, if psychology is a science comparable to physics or chemistry, it should definitely matter to practitioners of this science whether a brain or a computer is carrying out an algorithm.

Searle (1992) argues that the computer analogy is not only misleading, it is also incorrect and incoherent. As I noted above, a basic assumption of this analogy is that a particular algorithm can be carried out on a potentially infinite number of physical mechanisms. For example, one could add on one's fingers, on a calculator, on an abacus, and so on. Searle argues that "the multiple realizability of computationally equivalent processes in different physical media is not just a sign that the processes are abstract, but that they are not intrinsic to the system at all. They depend on an interpretation from the outside" (p. 209). In other words, people assign meaning to the inputs and the outputs of things such as calculators. Numbers and mathematical operations are not intrinsic to calculators because we could make the same transistor states and key presses correspond to words and other things, not just to numbers. But if the brain causes cognition (as most people think it does), then cognition *is* an intrinsic property of the brain in the way computation seems not to be. As such, cognition is more like features of the world such as the molecular structure of substances (e.g., H_2O for water) or the shape and color of common objects (e.g., the roundness of an orange). Computation, in contrast, is more like features such as "nice day for a picnic" which require an observer to assign this property to the world (Searle, 1992). Take away the observer and the latter feature would not exist.

Argument 2: The Explanatory Vocabulary Account

Scientific theories are said to "carve nature at its joints" (Pylyshyn, 1984; Kosslyn & Koenig, 1992). Individual sciences, however, carve nature at different levels of analysis and explain different types of phenomena. To illustrate, imagine a situation in which a physicist, a biologist, and a psychologist all attend the same baseball game. During a particular inning, the pitcher throws a curve ball and strikes a batter out. If someone were to ask "Why did he throw a curve ball?," the psychologist could provide a satisfactory answer to this question by making use of mainstream psychological constructs such as knowledge and desires (e.g., "He *wanted* to strike him out and *knew* that the batter was not very good at hitting curve balls"). In contrast, neither the physicist nor the biologist could provide a satisfactory answer using mainstream constructs from physics or biology. For example, the physicist would have to say something like "Air currents operating over the laces caused the ball to curve . . . ," while the biologist would have to say something like "Neural impulses traveled down his arm, causing a contraction in his right arm muscle. . . . " Note that such answers tell us why the ball curves and how a human body can move to produce a curve ball, but they do not directly answer the question asked above. In a sense, then, there are certain questions that only a psychological theorist could answer in the manner intended. As such, anyone who tried to answer psychological questions with a biological (or even quasi-biological) vocabulary would end up providing an inadequate answer (Pylyshyn, 1984; Putnam, 1973).

Although this account seems reasonable, note that it assumes that someone would try to provide a neurological answer to a psychological question. Neuroscience does not provide answers to questions such as

"Why did he throw a curve ball?," but rather to questions that *follow up* on psychological answers. For example, after learning about Baddeley's (1999) claim that there are two kinds of working memory systems, spatial and verbal, a neuroscientist might ask, "I wonder if there are regions of the brain that correspond to these two types of memory?" Similarly, after learning that gifted children seem to solve math problems more proficiently than nongifted children, a neuroscientifically oriented researcher might wonder whether math knowledge is represented differently in the brains of gifted and nongifted students. Thus, neuroscientific questions extend well beyond questions having to do with the brain's ability to carry out some function. To suggest that neuroscience can only answer such "how" questions is misleading.

Note further that the explanatory vocabulary account was originally proposed as a argument against reductionism (not against the utility of asking neuroscientific questions). Reductionist philosophers argue that the laws of so-called higher level sciences such as psychology and sociology are reducible to the lower level sciences such as biology, chemistry, and physics (Putnam, 1973). As such, reductionists argue that the only reason we use psychological vocabulary terms is because we have not quite figured out the biology. By showing that the psychological explanatory vocabulary is indispensable, the anti-reductionists show that psychology is not reducible to biology.

At this point, it should be noted that there is an important difference between (1) being interested in the implications of neuroscientific research for psychological theories and (2) wanting to replace a vague psychological terminology with a more precise biological vocabulary. Whereas the latter approach is reductionistic, the former approach is not because the focus of interest is the interface between two sciences that continue to maintain their separate existences and integrity. As will become clear, I adopt and promote the interface approach in this book. In essence, then, there is no basis to the claim that an interest in the brain necessarily makes one reductionistic.

Argument 3: Too Little Is Known about the Brain

Some scholars have suggested that neuroscientific research is not terribly informative at present because the data are still somewhat tentative and basic. If this claim is true, then psychologists have two choices: they can either wait until more neuroscientific information comes in before constructing a model of cognition, or they can forge ahead on their own without considering the biological plausibility of their models. Several prominent individuals have argued that the latter course of action is the better way to go (Neisser, 1967; Simon, 1996). Not surprisingly, many of these same individuals advocated the computational theory of mind.

Although this "forge ahead alone" approach seems reasonable, closer analysis suggests that it may be somewhat unrealistic and could likely lead to a number of mistakes. To see this, consider the following analogy. Imagine that a young couple paid $2,000 to an architect to design a house for them but forgot to tell the architect about certain important constraints on the possible solutions (e.g., the house has to be less than 2,800 square feet, strong enough to survive an earthquake, etc.). In the real world, a good architect would probably inquire about these constraints before spending time on a design, but assume that in this case he or she did not. In this hypothetical situation, we can see that an architect who is uninformed about the constraints could easily design a house that is all wrong for the couple. If the couple has to pay $2,000 for each design, their money (and the architect's time) would be wasted on each erroneous solution.

In the case of a psychologist, there are some very real biological constraints on the possible solutions to the problem of designing an accurate model of cognition (Sejnowski & Churchland, 1989). As such, theorists who ignore these constraints could very well make a number of errors and be wasting their time. But does this mean that cognitive theorists need to wait and do nothing until more knowledge about the brain comes in? A little reflection reveals that they do not. At the very least, cognitive researchers should conduct studies to determine the kinds of elementary operations that might be carried out in specific regions of the brain (Posner & Raichle, 1994; Stanovich, 1998). Should regions corresponding to these elementary operations be discovered, the model proposed by cognitive researchers gains support. In effect, cognitive researchers provide the "road map" for potentially exciting and corroborating neuroscientific studies (Byrnes & Fox, 1998).

In addition, studies that originate from the perspective of neuroscience can reveal serendipitous findings that would not have been anticipated by the cognitive researcher (Byrnes & Fox, 1998). For example, we might learn that a particular region of the brain is highly active whenever someone is either experiencing negative emotions *or* speaking fluently (Posner & Raichle, 1994). The question then becomes, Why might these two seemingly disparate mental functions activate the same region of the brain? Are they somehow related? By being informed of such unanticipated findings, cognitive theory can be further enhanced. Thus, cognitive researchers should not forge ahead on their own. Rather, they should engage in active collaboration and communication with colleagues in the neurosciences.

Summary

Several compelling arguments can be used by psychologists or educators to bolster their case that they need not learn more about the brain. However, there is good reason to think that these arguments are based on misleading assumptions. My central premise in this book is that neuroscientific evidence is clearly relevant to the extent that it (1) corroborates (or refutes) contemporary models of cognition and learning, and (2) generates surprising findings that would not have been anticipated if one were to rely solely on contemporary psychological theories that lack a neuroscientific emphasis.

SOME ESSENTIAL NEUROSCIENTIFIC TERMS AND BRAIN STRUCTURES

Much of the research summarized in this book focuses on the location of elementary cognitive operations in the brain (e.g., the ability to associate printed words with sounds; see Chapter 6). Although some readers would probably prefer language such as "a little bulge in the cerebral cortex slightly above and behind your right ear" to describe such locations, the more conventional terms used by neuroscientists (in this case, the left angular gyrus) will be employed in the present book. Learning these terms is a little like learning the vocabulary of a foreign language, but the reader will find the former task fairly easy because the number of neuroscientific terms that have to be mastered to comprehend core ideas is quite limited. In addition, many of these terms recur in multiple chapters.

Neuroanatomists subdivide brain structures in several different ways. One approach is to group structures according to their presence versus absence (or relative size) in certain species, and to link the emergence of certain structures (e.g., large frontal lobes) to important events in evolutionary history (e.g., symbolic communication and tool use). This approach has led to the use of such expressions as "old brain" (i.e., structures that have been around for quite a long time) and "new brain" (i.e., structures that appeared most recently in evolutionary history). Another approach is to group structures according to types of brain tissue (e.g., gray matter vs. white matter; a preponderance of glial cells vs. pyramidal cells; etc.). A third approach is to group structures in terms of their linkage to early events in prenatal brain development. For the present purposes, I shall truncate all such analyses considerably by primarily subdividing the brain in terms of

(1) the cerebral cortex, (2) several important subcortical structures, and (3) Brodmann areas.

Cerebral Cortex

The *cerebral cortex* is the uppermost structure in the brain and has a highly convoluted appearance. The folds exist because the surface area of the cortex (about 2,400 square centimeters) is too large to fit within the space allotted to it in the skull (Johnson, 1997). The bulging part of each fold is called a *gyrus* (plural, *gyri*); the grooves that run between gyri are called sulci (singular *sulcus*). As we shall see in subsequent chapters, the cerebral cortex is primarily involved in the processing of sensory information (e.g., visual, auditory, etc.), the control of movements, and the storage of experiences (i.e., learning and memory). Figure 1.1 shows the cerebral cortex as well as its four lobes (i.e., *frontal, temporal, parietal*, and *occipital*). This side (or *lateral*) view of the brain shows what it would look like if a person were looking to the reader's left and his or her skull were removed. Hence, the frontal lobes lie just behind a person's forehead. The right side of the brain has a similar appearance and is also subdivided into the same four lobes. A top view would show that the cerebral cortex is divided into two halves, or *hemispheres* (right and left). So the left frontal, left temporal, left parietal, and left occipital lobes all lie in (and comprise) the left hemisphere. The right frontal, right temporal, right parietal, and right occipital lobes all lie in (and comprise) the right hemisphere.

At this point, it would be useful to introduce some of the directional terminology found in the neuroscientific literature. This terminology was introduced by scientists and physicians in order to create an efficient and precise way to indicate the location of such things as tumors and lesions. To see the need for efficiency, note how cumbersome it would be to always preface one's description of a location with phrases such as "Imagine that a patient were facing to your left. . . . " To see the need for precision, a surgeon would need to know more than the hemisphere that contains a tumor; he or she would also need to know the lobe (e.g., frontal) and location within the lobe (e.g., near the top of the frontal lobe, 3 inches from the midline that separates the hemispheres). The convention developed by scientists combines a top-to-bottom orientation with a face-to-back-of-head orientation. Locations found near the top of some structure are said to be *superior* (and also *dorsal*, like the "dorsal fin" on the back of a dolphin). Those lying near the bottom are called *inferior* (and also *ventral*). As for the front-to-back orientation, structures lying more toward one's face are called *anterior* (also *rostral*; *rostrum* is

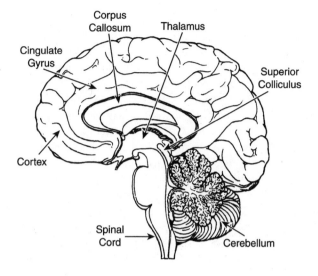

FIGURE 1.2. Sagittal view to review important subcortical structures.

the frontal lobe (associated with speech and verbal working memory), Areas 22 and 42 in the temporal lobe (associated with auditory processing), Areas 40 and 39 in the parietal lobe (associated with spatial working memory and phonetic processing), and Areas 17, 18, and 19 in the occipital lobes (associated with visual processing). Area 44 is also known as *Broca's area* and is well known for being associated with ex-

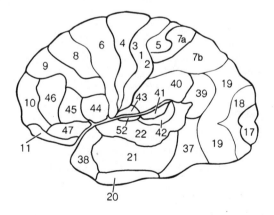

FIGURE 1.3. Brodmann areas of the cortex.

pressive aphasia (the inability to produce speech). Another type of receptive aphasia (*Wernicke's aphasia*) occurs when there is damage to both Areas 22 and 39. Here, an individual loses the ability to understand either visual or auditory language input. One other important area worth noting is the *dorsolateral prefrontal cortex* (DLPC) which mainly involves a gyrus that lies superior to Areas 44 and 45. Among other things, the DLPC has been implicated in tasks involving working memory and behavioral inhibition (Goldman-Rakic, 1994).

As one further way to organize the anatomical information that appears in this book, consider the matrix in Table 1.1. It lists key brain structures down the left column and the definition, location, and some of the presumed functions of these structures down the remaining columns. Also, the reader can refer to the Glossary of terms at the end of this book. In my view, the best way to gain facility over these terms is to encounter them in context in subsequent chapters and refer to sections of this chapter, figures, and the Glossary as semantic memory aides. The reader will find that he or she needs the memory prompts less and less as he or she progresses through this book.

NEUROSCIENTIFIC RESEARCH METHODS AND THEIR LIMITATIONS

Earlier, I suggested that neuroscientists tend to ask different questions than psychologists. Whereas a typical psychological question might be "How many different types of memory are there?," a typical neuroscientific question might be "Which regions of the brain are associated with spatial memory?" To answer questions such as the latter, neuroscientists have relied on four main methodological techniques: (1) case studies of brain-injured individuals, (2) surgical techniques with animals, (3) neuroimagining, and (4) gross electrical recording. In what follows, each of these approaches will be described and critiqued in turn.

Case Studies of Brain-Injured Individuals

Researchers who analyze the effect of brain lesions on cognitive functions are called "cognitive neuropsychologists" (McCarthy & Warrington, 1990; Kosslyn & Koenig, 1992). Through a careful analysis of case studies, cognitive neuropsychologists have attempted to link specific regions of the brain with specific cognitive processes. As I noted earlier, for example, individuals who have lesions in the third frontal convolution of the left hemisphere (i.e., the Broca area, or

TABLE 1.1. An Organizational Matrix of Brain Structures

Structure	Location	Relevant functions
Cerebral cortex	Top layer of brain tissue subdivided into lobes	See lobes for specifics
Frontal lobes	Anterior portions of cortex behind forehead	Certain verbal and reading skills, aspects of memory, attentional vigilance, stress, arousal, inhibition, emotional processing, reasoning, math skills
Temporal lobes	Lateral portions of cortex behind ears and side of head	Processing of auditory information, aspects of memory, emotional reactions, math skills, dyslexia
Parietal lobes	Superior, posterior portions of the cortex	Aspects of memory, aspects of attention, math skills
Occipital lobes	Posterior portion of cortex behind back of head	Visual processing, spatial working memory
Subcortical structures		
Thalamus	Inside middle of brain	Rote memory, aspects of attention, arousal, emotional responding
Superior colliculus	Posterior and inferior to thalamus	Eye movements, visual attention
Corpus callosum	Superior to thalamus	Fibers that allow communication between hemispheres
Cingulate gyrus	Superior to corpus callosum	Anterior portion used when people engage in many cognitive tasks
Cerebellum	Inferior and posterior to temporal and occipital lobes	Motor coordination, balance, conditioning, certain verbal and visual tasks

Note. There are many other structures in the brain but most have not been implicated in the processes described in this book (e.g., memory); also, the structures in the table have other functions as well.

Brodmann Area 44) often lose the ability to utter words but can still understand what is being said to them. In contrast, individuals who sustain damage to the Wernicke area (located near the temporal–parietal junction in the left hemisphere) can utter words but do not understand what is said to them and often speak nonsensically (McCarthy & Warrington, 1990). Such patterns of selective losses in distinct domains have been called *double dissociations*. In addition to studying the natural occurrence of lesions in humans, researchers have gained insight into regional functions by examining what happens as the brain is progressively anesthetized prior to an operation and what happens after the corpus callosum is severed to relieve epilepsy (Squire, 1987; McCarthy & Warrington, 1990).

Whereas the analysis of brain injuries and postoperative performance has revealed much about the nature of cognitive processes such as reading or memory, this approach has several important limitations. In the first place, techniques such as single-unit recording and surgery have revealed that specific components of a larger skill (e.g., detecting the orientation of lines) are related to rather small regions of the brain. Most naturally occurring lesions affect multiple small regions at once (Kosslyn & Koenig, 1992; Squire, 1987). Second, if damage to a region impairs a specific behavior, it cannot be assumed with certainty that the region (or hemisphere) in question controls that behavior. To illustrate this point, Kosslyn and Intriligator (1992) note that whereas removing a resistor from a radio may make it howl, the resistor is not a "howl suppressor." Third, damage to an area usually does not completely eliminate a skill: it merely lowers performance substantially. If there were a one-to-one correspondence between a region and a skill, logic dictates that the skill should entirely disappear following extensive damage. Fourth, there is considerable individual variability in the locations that cause a specific deficit in people (McCarthy & Warrington, 1990). For example, whereas frontal lobe damage reduces the ability to name objects in some patients, temporal lobe damage does so in others.

In the past few years, researchers have attempted to produce "virtual" or temporary lesions using a technique called *transcranial magnetic stimulation* (TMS). In TMS, a large current is passed through a hand-held coil that generates a magnetic field (Walsh & Rushworth, 1999). The magnetic field passes through the scalp and penetrates cortical tissue. The magnetic field effects the cortex by producing neural activity. When a region of the brain is actively performing some task (e.g., speech), a repetitive series of pulses can cause a disruption of that task (e.g., slurred speech). Moreover, pulses applied to the motor cortex can cause an individual to engage in a reflexive movement of particular digits or limbs (depending on where it is applied). One can, then, create a functional map of the cortex based on the skills that are executed or disrupted when a pulse is applied to various areas. In contrast to studies of naturally occurring injuries, moreover, TMS seems to have much better spatial resolution. For example, the apparent function of scalp areas as close as 1 centimeter apart can be distinguished. TMS is not without its problems, however. It can sometimes cause seizures, migraine headaches, nausea, and emotional responses (e.g., crying).

Surgical Techniques with Animals

A variety of experimental techniques that could not ethically be used with humans have been used with animals to study brain function. For example, there are surgical techniques such as (1) making incisions in, or removing portions of, the brains of animals in specific locations to observe losses of function; and (2) transplanting brain tissues in animal fetuses to see if the transplated tissues make appropriate neural connections (Goldman-Rakic, 1986; Johnson, 1993; Squire, 1987). In addition, substances (e.g., hormones, neurotransmitter blockers, etc.) can be inserted into animal brains to see their effect on learning or brain morphology (Squire, 1987; Halpern, 1992). Third, the temperature of portions of animal brains can be lowered to produce temporary disabilities. Fourth, there is single-unit recording, which involves the insertion of a microelectrode into the brain to record local extracellular potentials (Recanzone, Schreiner, & Merzenich, 1993; Sejnowski & Churchland, 1989). Hubel and Wiesel (1962) used single-unit recording when they performed their groundbreaking work on the neuroanatomy of vision in cats, and Goldman-Rakic (1994) has used it to map out the circuitry connecting the frontal and parietal lobes of monkeys. Finally, there are environmental enrichment studies in which animals are reared in different environments and then sacrificed to study the effect of enrichment on neuronal growth and synaptogenesis in the brain (Greenough, Black, & Wallace, 1987).

The major advantage of all these approaches is that researchers can precisely manipulate or closely monitor just those brain regions of interest. In effect, they have been able to experimentally alter "nature" instead of relying on correlational analyses (as has to be done with humans). Although much has been learned from these studies using these methods, limitations restrict what psychologists or educators can infer from them. First, behaviors in animals are far less flexible than behaviors in humans (Johnson, 1997; Vygotsky, 1978). For example, whereas an injection of sex hormones might prompt an animal to reflexively engage in a single, very specific mating behavior, it might prompt a human to consider engaging in a wide class of nonspecific sexual behaviors (in the same way that hormones responsible for hunger would make one feel hungry but not specify what one should eat). Second, humans possess higher order skills that animals lack (e.g., reading). Hence, animals cannot be used to study these processes. Third, the locations of certain processes differ in animals and humans. For example, whereas working memory seems to be associated with the hippocampus in rats, working memory seems to be associated with other regions (e.g., the frontal and parietal lobes) in humans (Goldman-Rakic, 1994; Squire, 1987). Fourth, brain maturational processes differ among species. For example, whereas synaptic density in infant monkeys and humans is 75–95% above the adult value, the infant value for kittens is only 50% above the adult value and that for rats is only 10% above the adult value (Huttenlocher, 1993). Combined with data suggesting that there is less neuronal death in some species than in others, it seems that more complex cortical systems rely more on synapse elimination than on preprogrammed neuronal death as infant brains are transformed into adult brains (Huttenlocher, 1993; see Chapter 2 for more on brain development). All of these differences in conjunction with important interconnectivity differences among species mean that what is true for an animal brain may not be true for a human brain.

As I describe later, certain claims regarding neural plasticity, the genetic basis of gender differences, and experiential effects on brain structure have all been based on animal studies. The aforementioned limitations of these studies mean that the reader should interpret such findings with appropriate caution.

Neuroimaging Techniques

Computed tomography (CT) and magnetic resonance imaging (MRI) help determine the location of lesions and tumors in the brain as well as reveal the size and shape of brain regions (Sejnowski & Churchland, 1989). Prior to the development of these techniques, researchers had to rely on surgery or postmortem studies to discover the precise location and extent of injury or malformations. But CT and older versions of MRI are limited because they cannot reveal the locations of the brain that are active when someone tries to perform a task. In contrast, functional magnetic resonance imaging (fMRI) and positron emission tomography (PET) can reveal active areas (Cherry & Phelps, 1996; Cohen, 1996).

All types of MRI (including fMRI) utilize the natural magnetic properties of molecular particles in substances. Similar to simple household magnets, the molecules of many substances (e.g., water) have positive and negative poles. When a strong magnetic field is passed over these molecules, most tend to align themselves in the direction of the field. When the magnetic field is turned off and a pulse of harmless radiation is directed toward the aligned molecules, some of the molecules reverse their polar orientation and give off a small amount of energy. This energy can be detected and used to create a visual image of the substance in question (e.g., a slice of brain tissue). fMRI makes use of differences in the magnetic properties of different substances to create images of active areas of the brain. For example, images can be enhanced by injecting contrast agents into a person's bloodstream. The contrast agents alter the magnetic resonance (MR) signal of water molecules in the cranial vasculature such that these signals are distinct from the MR signals of water molecules in brain tissues (Moonen, 1995). Another approach is to rely on differences in the magnetic properties of oxygenated and deoxygenated hemoglobin (e.g., Engel et al., 1994). All such fMRI techniques rely on the assumption that shifts in blood flow correlate with shifts in mental activity. That is, it is assumed that blood is sent to areas of the brain that are active during a task.

In recent years, fMRI has become the method of choice for three reasons: (1) it has excellent spatial and temporal resolution (i.e., it identifies the location of activity within a few millimeters and records the activity a few seconds after it occurs); (2) subjects are not exposed to ionizing radiation; and (3) an individual subject can be studied repeatedly (Cohen, 1996; Moonen, 1995). The third benefit means that researchers can avoid the intersubject averaging of signals that is required with PET (see below). Nevertheless, the cost of the procedure can be prohibitive because very powerful magnets are needed to achieve an adequate signal. In addition, people are asked to perform tasks as they lie on their backs in a tubular chamber that makes a very loud clanging sound and often causes claustrophobic reactions. Together, these first two problems explain why most fMRI studies seem to have fewer than 10 people per experimental group. A third problem derives from the use of the so-called subtraction technique to identify localized areas of high activity for a particular task. Here, a resultant image is computed after a number of t-tests are performed to identify significant differences in the pixels of a pair of images (Casey et al., 1996). If the significance levels of these t-tests are not adjusted to compensate for the large number of tests performed, errors of statistical inference could be made. Another problem with the subtraction technique is that one can never be certain that the subtraction really isolates the skill in question (Posner & Raichle, 1994).

A fourth problem derives from individual differences in the size and convolution patterns of brains (Goldman-Rakic, 1994; Talairach & Tournoux, 1988). In one person, the Broca area may be 8 centimeters from the top of the cortex and 3 centimeters to the left of the central sulcus (the sulcus that separates the frontal and parietal lobes). In another person with a smaller brain, however, the Broca area may be only 6 centimeters from the top and only 2 centimeters to the left of the central sulcus. Such differences in size mean that a "map" constructed for one person could not be used to identify active locations in the brain of the other person. Doing so would be like using the map of Texas to locate cities in Rhode Island. Most studies that use fMRI resort to using mathematical algorithms to put everyone on comparable scales. The algorithms are based on the idea of using a three-dimensional proportional grid system developed by Talairach and Tournoux (1988). This system, which exploits certain commonalities in the brains of all people (e.g., the fact that the central sulcus nearly always falls within 2 centimeters of a focal vertical line in the system), is slowly replacing the use of Brodmann areas in the literature. But it should be noted that the mathematical conversions required in this new system could lead to inaccuracies in the placement of active areas.

The fifth problem with fMRI pertains to the fact that a number of unresolved issues make interpretation of MR signals difficult. For example, when one attempts to detect signals from hemoglobin in a person's blood, the increase in fMRI signals that seemingly accompany neural activity is caused by a *decrease* in deoxyhemoglobin (Moonen, 1995). A decrease in the concentration of deoxyhemoglobin is associated with a variety of physiological events, and it is not yet clear which of these events causes the decrease in deoxyhemoglobin. Until this ambiguity is clarified, it cannot be said with certainty that changes in MRI signals in a region definitely reflect increased neural activity in that region.

Turning now to PET, the basic procedure involves injecting a radioactive substance (e.g., an isotope of oxygen or fluorine) into the bloodstream. Advocates of PET assume that more active areas of the brain use more nutrients and oxygen than less active areas, so the more active areas will have more blood flow, and will therefore show a higher concentration of the isotope. The PET scanner records the positions of the isotope in the brain as an individual solves a task. High concentrations of the isotope show up on the computed image of the brain as dense areas of a particular color (e.g., red). For example, if a subject is asked to give the meaning of a word and the PET apparatus computes a dense area of red for a region near the inferior left frontal gyrus, researchers might infer that the inferior frontal gyrus is associated with semantic analysis.

The major problems of PET scanning include the expense and availability of the equipment, and the hazards associated with radioactive isotopes. As with fMRI, these problems often restrict sample size to less than 10 per group (e.g., eight brain-injured subjects and eight controls). Consequently, there is reason to be concerned about the reliability of the statistical inferences that one could draw from such studies. In addition, when the authors report their findings, they often average levels and areas of activity across trials and subjects. This approach will obscure individual differences in activity with respect to locations and give the impression that performance is more localized than research with lesions would suggest. For example, when activation is averaged during semantic processing, one may find that areas of the left frontal lobe are highly active. This does not mean, however, that all subjects show high levels of activation for that area. Finally, there is a problem of temporal resolution in PET scans. In some cases, activity must be averaged over 45 minutes, but a given task may take less than 1 second to perform (Sejnowski & Churchland, 1989). The latter problem can be somewhat alleviated by using some of the newer isotopes with short half-lives (e.g., oxygen-15 with a half-life of 2 minutes), but these shorter half-lives are still much longer than the time required to perform many tasks.

Gross Electrical Recording

The electroencephalogram (EEG) is a recording of electrical activity from the scalp that has been very useful for determining general regions of the brain that are specialized for specific modalities such as speech perception and bodily sensations (Sejnowski & Churchland, 1989). In addition, a specific component of the EEG called the event-related potential (ERP) has been linked to cognitive processing. For example, P300 is an ERP that occurs about 300 milliseconds after the introduction of an unexpected stimulus (e.g., a loud tone). Another ERP called N400 often occurs when a subject encounters a semantic incongruity (Kutas & Van Petten, 1988). The "P" and the "N" in these labels refer to either a peak (P for positive component) or a valley (N for negative component) in the printed wave-like output of the EEG.

The three major benefits of using EEGs and ERPs are that (1) the approach is noninvasive; (2) it can be used on alert, normal human subjects (including infants; see, e.g., Fox & Bell, 1990); and (3) it provides a better temporal resolution between underlying neurophysiology and behavior than other techniques such as PET and fMRI (Gevins, 1996). The major problem with EEG recording is that it "is a composite signal from volume conduction in many different parts of the brain, and it is far from clear what a signal means in terms of how neurons in the relevant networks are behaving" (Sejnowski & Churchland, 1989, p. 332). For example, P300 seems to have cortical and subcortical components. Whereas electrodes can be inserted in the brain to clarify the source of activity, there are obvious problems with attempting this technique with humans. Thus, there is always a degree of uncertainty about the precise brain locations that are active during a task when one uses an EEG, even when 64 electrodes are used (Gevins, 1996). In addition, individual differences in skull thickness and cell densities that may be confounded with task processing variables may obscure the meaning of the output. Also, recordings can only be made from cells that are aligned in a particular orientation. In the brain, cells are aligned in several orientations (see Chapter 2). Finally, the advantage in temporal resolution that EEGs once had over PETs and MRIs is getting smaller over time as the latter techniques have been improved (Gevins, 1996).

Summary

Overall, then, each of the approaches has its strengths and weaknesses. In order to avoid inappropriate inferences about structure–function relations, it is important to recognize the limitations of all these approaches and to avoid using the evidence from a single approach as unequivocal support for a particular claim. The most defensible approach is to make an inference about structure–function relations only when (1) *multiple* neuropsychological methods (e.g., lesions in humans, PET scans in humans, and animal studies) support a claim and (2) this claim squares with what has been found in traditional psychological experiments (Kosslyn & Koenig, 1992; Posner, Petersen, Fox, & Raichle, 1988; Sejnowski & Churchland, 1989). There is great excitement about the power of newer approaches (e.g., fMRI, TMS), and this excitement seems to prompt many to accept the findings without regard for the limitations of the methods. The reader should recognize that some of the claims made in such studies (e.g., about the location of functions) may well be discredited in the future as the methods in neuroscience mature and more is learned about the meaning of physiological signals.

One interesting development to watch is the use of two neuroscientific approaches in the same study. For example, some researchers are using PET combined with MRI to gain more precision in the localization of performance. Others are combining PET with 64-channel EEG to simultaneously note locations and temporal phases of performance (Posner, 1997). Using the latter technique, researchers have revealed activation patterns suggesting that readers seem to process written words in three steps: orthography first, then sound, then meaning.

SUMMARY AND PREVIEW OF REMAINING CHAPTERS

As I noted earlier, the goal of the present chapter was to provide an interpretive context for the chapters that follow. The arguments against the relevance of brain research (reviewed in the first section) and the limitations of neuroscientific methods (reviewed in the third section) were provided in order to engender a healthy sense of skepticism in the reader. By "healthy sense of skepticism," I mean an attitude that falls midway along a continuum of belief that ranges between complete dismissal of neuroscientific evidence and uncritical acceptance of it, as illustrated below:

|---------------------------------X----------------------------------|

| Complete | Realistic | Uncritical |
| Dismissal | Inferences | Acceptance |

The second section on neuroscientific vocabulary and the Glossary were written to serve as reference material that can be consulted as the need may be.

In Chapter 2, the processes of brain development are described. At issue is the manner in which intrinsic (e.g., genes) and extrinsic factors (e.g., experience) work together to produce a person's brain during development. In Chapters 3, 4, 5, 6, and 7, the psychological and neuroscientific perspectives on memory, attention, emotion, reading, and math skills, respectively, are described and compared. The goal in each case is to determine the extent to which the psychological and neuroscientific perspectives on these processes overlap. In addition, the instructional implications of these perspectives are also considered. In the final chapter, the goal is to revisit, integrate, and draw the implications of the research presented in Chapters 2 to 7.

CHAPTER 2

Brain Development

It has often been said that the best way to understand a finished product is to consider how it has been constructed over time (e.g., Vygotsky, 1978). Most of the chapters in this book are concerned with multiple aspects of a "finished" adult brain (e.g., the correlation between specific brain areas and specific cognitive functions). In the present chapter, the focus is on the processes by which this adult brain is progressively constructed during development.

By way of a preview, it is important to note that each of our brains has a specific *cytoarchitecture*, that is, it contains a certain number of neurons that are connected to each other in particular ways. Inasmuch as this cytoarchitecture is the computational foundation of our ability to think and to reason, scientists have often wondered whether talented individuals differ from less talented individuals in terms of the number of neurons in their brain and the interconnections among these neurons. They have also tried to determine the extent to which a person's cytoarchitecture is determined by his or her genes. Although brain science has not advanced enough to know whether there is, in fact, a correlation between certain cytoarchitectures and talent, it has advanced enough to be able to say something about the role of genetics in the construction of individual brains. The goal of the present chapter is to present information relevant to the latter issue and related issues.

In the first section of this chapter, the notion of cytoarchitecture is explored further as a means of laying the groundwork for subsequent sections. Then, consideration is given to the processes by which this cytoarchitecture is constructed during prenatal and postnatal development. Finally, the factors that facilitate or hinder optimal brain development are discussed.

FURTHER EXPLORATIONS OF CYTOARCHITECTURE: CELL TYPES AND BRAIN LAYERS

Throughout this book, we shall see how specific cognitive operations (e.g., recognizing letter patterns) are localized in specific areas of the cortex (e.g., circuits within the occipital and parietal lobes). In addition to this *areal* organization, the cortex also has a characteristic *laminar* organization (i.e., layers that extend deeper into the brain). A prerequisite to understanding the latter type of organization is to recognize that the brain contains a number of different types of cells that fall into two broad classes: *glial cells* and *neurons*. Glial cells are far more numerous than neurons, but they do not seem to play a role in the processing of information (as far as scientists know). Instead, they serve a number of other important functions including (1) providing firmness and structure to the brain, (2) forming the myelin sheath that surrounds the axons of long neurons and speeds up their firing, (3) providing a "scaffold" for neurons to latch onto during the process of cell migration (see below), and (4) taking up and removing some of the chemical transmitters that are released during synaptic transmission (Kandel, 1991).

Neurons, in contrast, do play a role in the processing of information. They come in a variety of types that differ in terms of their shape, patterns of connectivity, and the neurotransmitters they release. The shape dimension underlies the distinction between *pyramidal cells* (see Figure 2.1) and other types of cells (e.g., star-shaped cells called *stellate*

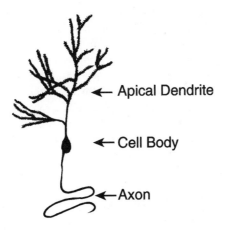

FIGURE 2.1. Basic structure of a pyramidal cell.

cells). The former comprise more than 80% of the neurons in the brain (Johnson, 1997; Moyer, 1980). The connectivity dimension underlies the distinction between excitatory and inhibitory neurons. The neuro-transmitter dimension allows one to distinguish between neurons that excrete dopamine, neurons that excrete gamma-aminobutyric acid (GABA), and neurons that excrete serotonin.

Scientists discovered these various aspects of neurons in the midst of examining microscopic slides of brain tissue. This microscopic approach also revealed the fact that the cortex is comprised of six horizontal layers that differ in terms of the morphology, density, and functional proper-ties of the neurons in them (Chenn, Braisted, McConnell, & O'Leary, 1997; Johnson, 1997). Layer 1 is the highest (most superior) layer and consists primarily of long, horizontal fibers that connect different re-gions of the cortex to each other. Layers 2 and 3 also contain horizontal fibers as well as small pyramidal cells that extend apical dendrites up-ward as well as collateral projections outward to neighbors. A dendrite is the branching portion of a neuron that receives neurotransmitters se-creted by presynaptic neurons (see Figure 2.1). Layer 4 is the terminal point for many input fibers from subcortical regions (e.g., the thalamus). These inputs primarily make contact with the large number of stellate cells found in Layer 4. Layers 5 and 6 are the most inferior (deepest) lay-ers that have a high concentration of large pyramidal cells that project long-distance, output fibers to important subcortical sites as well as api-cal dendrites that extend upward to Layers 4 and 1 (but not to Layers 2 and 3). Thus, all the layers contain neurons that make either horizontal connections with neurons in other layers, or vertical connections with neurons in the same layer (or both).

This laminar arrangement of cells is a defining characteristic of an adult brain. As such, it can be used to judge the relative maturity of chil-dren's brains at various ages. For example, a researcher may wish to consider whether 5-year-old children seem to have the same number of stellate cells in Layer 4 as adults (e.g., Huttenlocher, 1993). Similarly, re-searchers might consider whether the neurons in children's brains seem to make the same number of synaptic connections as the neurons in adults' brains. In the next section, these issues are considered further as the processes that create the laminar structure of the brain are explored.

SEVEN MAJOR PROCESSES OF BRAIN DEVELOPMENT

Prenatal development is often characterized in terms of structurally de-fined phases, that is, the boundaries of specific prenatal periods are set by the emergence of particular structural or anatomical features in an embryo or fetus (Purves & Lichtman, 1985). The period of the *zygote*, for example, begins when an ovum is fertilized by a sperm and concludes when cell divisions within the zygote create a structure called a *blastula* (a hollow sphere of cells). Soon thereafter, the cells on the surface of the blastula invaginate along an indentation and create a groove called the *primitive streak*. The latter process is called *gastrulation* because it creates a structure called a *gastrula*. Somewhat later, during a process called *neurulation*, two symmetrical, protruding folds of tissue emerge on the longitudinal surface of the gastrula, move closer together (like two ocean waves moving toward each other), and eventually fuse above the primitive streak to form the *neural tube*. One end of the neural tube eventually gives rise to the structures of the forebrain and the midbrain. The other end eventually gives rise to the spinal cord (Johnson, 1997; Moyer, 1980). The end that gives rise to the forebrain and the midbrain structures continues to develop and expand in such a way that a characteristic pattern of five convolutions and bulges appears by 5 weeks gestational age (imagine a partially inflated, shaped balloon attached to a straw). Whereas the most anterior bulge is eventually transformed into the cortex, the second-most anterior bulge is eventually transformed into structures such as the thalamus and the hypothalamus (Johnson, 1997).

Early on, scientists suspected that these bulges arose because the neural tube was manufacturing brain cells somewhere inside its walls. To confirm this suspicion, they used microscopic techniques to observe the formation of bulges *in vivo*. They found two regions within the neural tube (called *proliferative zones*) out of which brain cells emerged in rapid succession. Subsequent studies revealed that precursor cells within the zones produced approximately 100 generations of clones of themselves through mitotic division (Rakic, 1993). *Mitotic division* involves creating exact duplicates and splitting into two identical "daughter" cells with a full complement of DNA (as opposed to *meiosis*, which creates gametes with half the DNA of the parent cell). For some types of neuron, each precursor ends up producing 10,000 offspring cells. Given that the process of proliferation is largely over by the seventh prenatal month and that children's brains contain more than 10^{11} cells, it follows that the two proliferative zones must produce progenitors at an explosive rate of 250,000 cells per minute (Johnson, 1997; Purves & Lichtman, 1985)!

Subsequent research revealed a second major process besides *proliferation* that is instrumental in determining the eventual configuration of cells in an adult brain: *migration*. To understand migration, it is helpful to imagine a (coronal) cross-section of the neural tube that has concentric circles corresponding to various layers (similar to a bull's eye pattern). The proliferative zones lie near the innermost layer of the tube wall (close to the hollow of the tube or the target of the bull's eye). The neural tube expands in an outward, bulging manner because newly created cells migrate away from the proliferative zones to the outer layers of the tube wall. More specifically, as each generation of cells is produced through repeated cell division, they migrate farther and farther away from the inner wall (in an inside-out, or radial, progression). Hence, the cells that end up near the outer wall of the neural tube were some of the last ones produced during the process of proliferation. This outer layer is called the *cortical plate* because it ultimately becomes part of the cortex of a mature brain.

In vivo studies have revealed that neurons migrate to outer layers in one of two ways. In the first, newly created cells emerge from the proliferative zones and push older "siblings" away from the zones as they emerge (in the same way that an advancing crowd of protesters would push a line of police backward). In the second, newly created cells traverse along glial cells that are aligned in a perpendicular direction to the concentric layers of the tube (like spokes in a wheel). The glial cells secrete a substance to which the migrating cells adhere (Rakic, 1993) and the migrating cells themselves adhere to each other using recently discovered adhesion molecules (Edelman, 1992).

So far, I have described two processes that could produce a brain that has the right number of cells (proliferation) that are located in the right places (migration). Next, we have to consider how the brain manages to produce the various *types* of cells that are stereotypically distributed across the six layers of the cerebral cortex (as described above in the description of the laminar organization of the cortex). There are two ways that a developing brain could make sure that the right kind of cells (e.g., stellate cells) end up in the right layer (e.g., Layer 4). One way would be to transform progenitor cells into the right type (via genetic transcription processes) immediately after they are produced within the proliferative zones. According to this approach, a cell would "know" what kind of neuron it will become even before it migrates. The second way would be to withhold transforming the progenitor cell until after it migrates to a particular layer. In the latter approach, chemicals secreted by neighboring cells "inform" the migrated cell about what kind of cell it should become (Chenn et al., 1997). Recent experimental studies suggest that both of these processes seem to be involved in creating various types of neurons. In the absence of chemical signals from neighbors, postmitotic progenitors differentiate into one and only one type of cell. When these same cells are transplanted to atypical layers, however, they differentiate into cells typical for that layer.

The correlation between the birth date of a cell and its final laminar position suggests that a neuron's phenotype might be determined early (Chenn et al., 1997). As I noted above, there are two main classes of neurons in the cortex: pyramidal and nonpyramidal. Whereas the majority of pyramidal cells use excitatory amino acids as neurotransmitters, the majority of nonpyramidal neurons use inhibitory neurotransmitters (e.g., GABA). Moreover, whereas nonpyramidal cells are distributed uniformly across the six layers of the cortex, excitatory pyramidal neurons are only found in particular layers. Recent evidence suggests that local signals from neighbors have differing effects on neuronal specification, depending on when a cell was produced. For example, studies of regions that contain a large number of inhibitory neurons show that cells transplanted to that region during a certain phase of their development (the "S-phase") fail to become inhibitory. Cells transplanted after this phase, however, express inhibitory neurotransmitters (Chenn et al., 1997).

With differentiation processes added to the mix, we now have a brain that has the right number and the right type of cells located in the right layers. But to create a fully mature brain, several additional things have to happen. First, each brain cell has to grow in size and send projections to other cells. Second, these cells have to form synaptic connections with some of the cells to which they project. Third, an optimal numerical correspondence has to emerge between presynaptic and postsynaptic neurons. (Note: when two neurons are connected in a one-way chain by way of a synapse, the one earlier in the chain is called presynaptic; the next one to which it sends neurotransmitters is called postsynaptic). Finally, a myelin sheath has to form along the axons of many of the longer neurons. Let's examine each of these four processes a little further.

A fascinating aspect of neuronal growth processes is that neurons seem to seek out highly specific targets during their development. In experiments with animal brains, even when the targets of these projections are transplanted to atypical locations, the axons of the seeking neurons still find their targets (Chenn et al., 1997; Purves & Lichtman, 1985). Other evidence of neuronal specificity is the fact that there is a highly stereotyped pattern of lamina-specific axonal projections across individuals. For example, whereas Layer 5 neurons make long-distance projections to targets such as the spinal cord and the superior colliculus in most people, those in Layer 6 make long-distance projections to the thalamus (Chenn et al., 1997). Unlike the synaptic connections that form in response to experience (see later in this chapter and in Chapter 3), the stereotyped, laminar patterning of connections among neurons seems to be largely determined by genes (Chenn et al., 1997; Goodman & Tessier-Lavigne, 1997).

Although the evidence is still coming in, it would appear that a combination of factors explain how it is that neurons can find their genetically determined targets. The first thing to note is that axons solve the daunting task of finding long-distance targets by proceeding in small steps (Goodman & Tessier-Lavigne, 1997). That is, they project a small distance and leave behind a new portion of axon. At each point, they make use of both local cues (e.g., *chemoaffinity*, or attraction to certain "guidepost" cells along the way, as well as repulsion toward other cells), and long-distance cues (e.g., a steady increase in the concentration of neuronal growth factor [NGF] as the axon gets closer to the target). Then gradations of molecular guideposts along the surface of targets help individual axons recognize their targets.

Once the projected axons of neurons are in close proximity to other neurons, a correlation of activity patterns in these neurons promotes the formation of synapses. In other words, if two neurons are always active at the same times, they are likely to form a synapse with each other. If they are active at different times, however, they are unlikely to form synapses with each other. In the developing fetus, these activity patterns seem to be intrinsic and spontaneous (i.e., they are not caused by afferent stimulation from the environment that travels from sensory organs along pathways and registers ultimately in the brain; they fire in an unprovoked manner). The first sign that a synapse is forming is that the membranes of the presynaptic and postsynaptic cells thicken at the site of the synapse in response to recurrent activity. The second sign is that the tip of the axon changes in appearance from looking like a *growth cone* (i.e., a starburst) to looking like a *synaptic bouton* (an oval with a flat bottom; imagine a cloth bag of marbles tied at the top). Then, three other changes take place: (1) circular vesicles containing neurotransmitters appear near the edge of the bouton (imagine a row of dots along the bottom of the bag), (2) the synaptic cleft between the bouton and the surface of the postsynaptic neuron's dendrite widens somewhat (i.e., forms a narrow oval shape), and (3) glial cells encase the boutons. The net result of all these anatomical changes is that the information exchange between presynaptic and postsynaptic neurons can occur in a fast and efficient manner. From the standpoint of neuroscience, however, we need to know what a mature synapse looks like before we can say anything about changes in synapses that occur with age or experience. When a scientist counts the number of fully formed synapses in a region of a child's brain and in a region of an adult's brain, for example, he or she needs to be able to recognize a fully formed synapse.

In an adult brain, each of the approximately 10^{11} neurons makes 1,000 or more synaptic contacts with other neurons (Goodman & Tessier-Lavigne, 1997). In addition, these neurons tend to form contacts in a stereotypical manner. For example, some neurons form synapses only on dendritic spines, while others form synapses only on dendritic shafts (note: the spines are like circular leaves on a tree and the shafts are like branches). Early in development, however, this stereotyped patterning is not yet apparent and neurons make many more synaptic contacts than needed to create functional circuits for processing information. So, slides of brain tissue from a young child would reveal lots of synapses all over the neuron, while slides from an adult would reveal a stereotyped reduced pattern. One way that the overabundance of synapses is reduced with age (in many species) is through the death of neurons. A second way is through the process of axonal retraction. In the latter process, a presynaptic neuron literally retracts its axon away from the postsynaptic neuron (by shrinking in size; imagine a tree pulling back one of its branches away from a neighboring tree by making it smaller).

What causes neurons to die and why do surviving neurons retract their axons? Many scientists believe that both of these processes reflect the fact that neurons have to compete for substances called *trophic factors* that are secreted by activated postsynaptic neurons (Purves & Lichtman, 1985; Reichardt & Farinas, 1997). To explain cell death, they note that only some of the axonal projections that make contact with target neurons will succeed in obtaining enough trophic factors to survive. Those that survive and become activated at the same time as postsynaptic neurons tend to form stable synapses with these postsynaptic neurons. To explain axonal retraction, they note that sometimes neurons fail to get enough trophic factor from one site but succeed in getting enough from other sites. Instead of dying, these neurons simply retract their axons away from the unsupportive areas.

The net result of the competition for trophic factors is an optimum balance between a population of innervat*ing* neurons and a population of innervat*ed* neurons (i.e., a functional circuit that has the right number of each class of cells). Presumably, the initial oversupply of neurons and synapses emerged phylogenetically as an evolutionary adaptation to guard against possible problems that might arise as brains are being constructed. To see the utility of this oversupply, consider the following thought experiment. Imagine a species that had a brain that contained 300 functional circuits (one circuit for each of 300 cognitive operations). Next assume that each circuit must have 1,000 neurons configured in a

particular way to work properly (total = 300,000 neurons). Finally, assume the proliferative zones in this species produce exactly 300,000 cells
during development. A little reflection shows that a properly constructed
brain would only be constructed in this species if all of the following
happened during development: (1) all cells managed to migrate to the
right locations, (2) chemical signals from neighboring cells were detected
by the DNA transcription processes of all of the migrated cells, and (3)
the axons of all cells found their targets. In effect, a properly functioning
brain would only emerge if everything went right. But things often go
wrong in nature, so the biological strategy of producing exactly the
number of cells needed is obviously not the best way to go.

Shortly after the regressive processes of cell death and axonal retraction were discovered, scientists wondered whether all species relied
on these two processes to the same extent. Some recent evidence suggests
that lower order species (e.g., rats) seem to rely more on cell death than
higher order species (e.g., humans). The opposite seems to be true for
axonal retraction (Huttenlocher, 1993). However, this conclusion is
based on a few studies using postmortem techniques. Hence, more evidence needs to accumulate before strong statements can be made regarding interspecies differences in regressive processes.

The last two processes of brain development that should be discussed are *dendritic arborization* and *axonal myelination*. In addition to
growing in size (length and width), neurons also sprout new dendrites
(arborization) and acquire a myelin sheath along some of their axons.
The addition of new dendrites is thought to be the primary neural basis
of cognitive development (Quartz & Sejnowski, 1997). To get a vivid
image of arborization in your mind, neurons bathed in solutions that
foster sprouting look like "Chia pets" (those small ceramic animals that
one covers with a seed paste and waters)! Myelination, in contrast, is the
process of adding a fatty-acid coating (myelin) to the axon of some neurons to speed up their firing. Myelin adds considerable mass to the brain
beyond that produced by other types of growth. When the brain is finished maturing in late adolescence, it weighs four times as much as it did
at birth (Johnson, 1997). Of course, a brain is never really finished
changing in an absolute sense because there is a constant shifting of synaptic contacts with experience (see later in this chapter and in Chapter
3). In addition, the brain often shrinks in size for inactive, undernour-
ished individuals who live beyond age 80.

In a way, the foregoing discussion of brain development could be
transformed into a checklist for determining the state of development in
a child's brain. As I noted earlier, autopsies have been used to determine
the kinds of cells that normally appear in specific layers and the number

of synapses that form between cells in various regions of the brain. This "final state" can serve as the reference point for developmental comparisons. For example, one could ask, How many cells are present in Layer 4 at ages 1, 4, 7, 10, and 13? How many synapses per neuron are there, on average, in an adult brain and a child's brain? Moreover, once we know how things should "look" in an average adult brain that developed in an average environment, we can consider the effects of various substances or experiences on brain development. For example, we can compare the brains of individuals who smoked cigarettes for many years to those of individuals who did not smoke to see if there are differences in the number of neurons in particular regions, the number of synapses formed by these neurons, and so on. In the next section, we explore the latter theme more fully.

FACTORS AFFECTING BRAIN DEVELOPMENT

In the previous two sections, the focus was on describing the general characteristics of mature brains (e.g., the laminar organization of the cortex) as well as the processes that produce these general characteristics (e.g., migration). Such an approach reveals how all our brains are similar at a basic level. In the present section, the primary goal is to elucidate the factors that produce individual differences in brain structure (i.e., how all our brains are different). Five such factors will be described in turn: (1) genetics, (2) environmental stimulation, (3) nutrition, (4) steroids, and (5) teratogens.

Genetics

Long before scientists discovered genes, they knew that some intrinsic (i.e., nonenvironmental) factor was responsible for producing the large-scale physical differences that can be observed among species (Edelman, 1992). Today, we know that this intuition was clearly correct. The human brain looks very different from other mammalian brains (including our closest ape cousins) chiefly because of a difference in genetic instructions. But what about the more subtle differences in brain structure that arise between individuals of the same species (Goldman-Rakic, 1994; Talairach & Tournoux, 1988)? As I noted in Chapter 1, for example, the precise location of particular areas (e.g., Broca's area) differs slightly among individuals. Are these within-species differences also caused by genetic differences? In order to answer this question, I need to expand my earlier descriptions of proliferation, migration, and differentiation.

Then, we can consider the implications of this expanded analysis for two related lines of genetic research.

The most important variable that explains between-species differences in brain size is the length of the proliferation phase. As Finlay and Darlington (1995) note, an additional 17 doublings of precursor cells can yield 131,000 times the final number of neurons (roughly the difference in the number of neurons found between the brains of humans and shrews). How does a developing brain know when to stop proliferating cells? One possibility is that the proper number of mitotic divisions is encoded somewhere in the DNA of precursor cells. Another possibility is that precursor cells continue to double until they receive signals that enough cells have migrated to various locations in the brain (Chenn et al., 1997). Regardless of which of these possibilities turns out to be true, it should be clear that proliferation is largely under the control of genetic instructions.

The same could be said for migration and differentiation. Earlier in this chapter we saw how proliferated cells seem to be genetically destined to become particular types of cells and how they migrate to particular levels as soon as they leave the proliferative zones. However, we also saw that this predestination is not set in stone. Once again, signals from neighboring cells seem to play a role in determining the ultimate fate of particular cells. Thus, one could summarize the role of genetics so far by saying that genes largely constrain how things turn out, but there is a certain degree of protective flexibility built into the system.

One other point worth noting pertains to the probabilistic nature of migration. As cells migrate, they overlap, pass by, make contact with, and adhere to each other in a complex way (Edelman, 1992; Rakic, 1993). As a result, there is no way to know for sure where a given cell will end up when it migrates (Chenn et al., 1997). The stochastic, "bump-and-grind" quality of the migration process means that genetic instructions are not really analogous to blueprints. Whereas two houses built from the same blueprint would turn out to be identical (in terms of their size, location of rooms, etc.), two brains built from the same set of genetic instructions could be significantly different.

The latter point provides a nice segue to a second line of work that provides further insight into the role of genetics in brain development. Researchers who have conducted neuroscientific studies of twins have made two important findings. First, people who have exactly the same genetic instructions (i.e., monozygotic [MZ] twins) sometimes develop brains that are structurally different (Edelman, 1992; Segal, 1989; Steinmetz, Herzog, Schlaug, Huang, & Lanke, 1995). In fact, MZ twins have been found to develop brains that are mirror images of each other (e.g., one has a dominant left hemisphere while the other has a dominant right hemisphere). The other kind of twins, dizygotic or DZ twins, have different genes and are like two siblings except for the fact that they are born at the same time.

However, researchers have also found that there can be a relatively high concordance rate between MZ twins for disorders that are alleged to have a neurological basis. *Concordance rate* is the extent to which both of the twins have the same phenotype (i.e., both have the disorder or both lack the disorder). In a study of the genetic basis of reading disability, for example, DeFries, Gillis, and Wadsworth (1993) found that 53.5% of MZ twins were concordant for reading problems, compared to just 31.5% of dizygotic (DZ) twins. Note, however, that both of these concordance rates are considerably lower than 100%, which suggests that there is not a deterministic, one-to-one correspondence between genes and brain structure. Also, when DeFries et al. estimated the heritability of reading disability from their data, they found that genetics accounted for 44% of the variance in reading profiles, which means that 56% is explained by nongenetic factors. Later studies produced somewhat higher concordance rates and heretibility estimates (see, e.g., Knopik, Alarcon, & DeFries, 1997), but the overall findings are essentially the same. Since MZ twins are highly similar in terms of their height and weight (r = .97), it would appear that reading disability is probably not a product of proliferation problems. Rather, it would seem that reading problems arise from other aspects of brain development (e.g., formation of synapses, pruning of axons, etc.; see Chapter 7).

A final way to assess the relative importance of genes for brain development is to examine disorders such as Down syndrome in which there is a known linkage between specific genes and neurological pathology. Down syndrome (DS) or Trisomy 21 is the leading cause of mental retardation in the United States. It results from the nondisjunction of a portion of the 21st chromosome during meiosis, so that three copies of that portion are present in the cells of the affected individual instead of the usual two (Coyle, Oster-Granite, Reeves, & Gearhart, 1988; Hassold, Sherman, & Hunt, 1995). The presence of this extra genetic material produces a number of anatomical and health-related differences between individuals with DS and unimpaired individuals (Coyle et al., 1988; Kemper, 1988). Of particular interest here are the differences related to brain structure. Individuals with DS tend to have brains that are smaller and less developed than those of unimpaired children and adults. In addition, individuals with DS tend to have 33% fewer cortical neurons, less complex patterns of connectivity, reduced levels of myelin, and apical dendrites that are abnormal in appearance (e.g., with fewer spines and elongated necks). Taken together, these findings suggest that the extra genetic material probably interferes with the processes of proliferation, synaptogenesis, and myelination.

Although much more can be said about the role of genes in brain development, the preceding discussion of developmental processes (e.g., proliferation), twin research, and genetic disorders is sufficient for drawing several broad conclusions. First, it seems clear that certain changes in genetic instructions can lead to large-scale changes in brain volume and patterns of connectivity. For example, a 2% change in the amount of genetic material (e.g., shifting from 46 to 47 chromosomes) can produce a 33% difference in brain structure (e.g., the number of cortical neurons in the brains of persons with DS vs. unimpaired individuals). But even when people have the same genes, there is still a chance that they could have brains that differ somewhat in terms of their size, shape, and areal organization. The lack of one-to-one correspondence between genes and brain structure means that researchers should not assume that two individuals definitely have different genes simply because their brains are different in size or in organizational structure. Perhaps more to the point, researchers should not argue with certainty that two people have different brains because they have different genes (consider the case of identical twins), nor argue with certainty that two people must have the same genes because their brains seem to be anatomically identical (two unrelated people who share few genes could have identical brains).

Environmental Stimulation

In essence, then, we see that genes only partly explain why we have the brains that we do. The second factor that is instrumental in sculpting the brain is environmental stimulation. In order for animals to respond adaptively to their environment, they have to be able to form mental representations that match their experiences (Greenough, Black, & Wallace, 1987; Johnson, 1997). For example, they need to be able to recognize conspecifics (e.g., their mothers and their siblings), as well as to store new, adaptation-relevant experiences in memory (e.g., the fact that fire can burn). Many animals come into the world ready to learn such things, using a prewired circuitry that is closely aligned with their external sense organs.

The prewired circuitry consists of (1) *cortical neurons* that receive, process, and store input signals from the environment and (2) *afferent neurons* that bring these input signals to the brain from the various sensory organs. Postmortem studies reveal that the afferent neurons from particular sensory organs terminate in the same general regions for all people (e.g., Area V1 in the occipital lobes in the case of afferents coming from the eyes). By necessity, then, it would be expected that all people would process and store input signals from particular organs in roughly the same regions of the cortex (Johnson, 1997). But it is important to note that this areal organization is jointly a function of the preset location of afferent projections and environmental stimulation. Take away the afferents and we would not develop particular types of representations (e.g., visual representations of the people we know) in particular regions of the cortex (e.g., Area V1). Similarly, we would obviously not develop representations of events in the world without experiencing these events. Each of these counterfactual claims has been tested empirically.

For example, surgical studies with animals have shown that atypical cortical maps can be created by redirecting the input fibers that extend from the thalamus to new areas. For example, normally, a neural tract that carries visual information from the eyes projects upward and backward from the thalamus in the middle of the brain to Area V1 of the occipital lobe in the cortex (in the back of the head). Scientists have redirected this tract such that it projects to, say, the frontal lobe. They find that cells in the frontal lobe then process visual information the same way cells in the occipital lobe normally do! In addition, studies have shown that animals will create new projections and new representations in a cortical area even after some of the thalamic projections that normally project to that area have been severed (e.g., Recanzone et al., 1993). A similar type of plasticity has been observed in human infants who have suffered brain injury or had portions of their brains removed to relieve epilepsy (Johnson, 1997). Normally, the neural regions responsible for language skills are in the left hemisphere for most right-handed people. Infants who have had their left hemispheres removed to relieve constant seizures develop language areas in their remaining right hemispheres. Thus, whereas the laminar organization of the cortex seems to be largely intrinsically determined (i.e., preprogrammed by genes and unrelated to afferent stimulation that comes into the cortex), the areal organization seems to be jointly determined by preexisting projections and environmental input (Chenn et al., 1997; Johnson, 1997). To understand the latter point by analogy, imagine that the neural assemblies in the cortex that process faces are like employees of a credit card company who operate in their own cubicles. Imagine further that outside phone calls from their customers are analogous to afferent stimulation from the environment. The company could not do its business if someone (e.g., the boss) had not placed the workers there and hooked them up to phone lines and each other via a computer network. But their computer databases would all be empty if their customers never called in. Thus a functioning company requires both preset architectures ready to receive input and the input itself.

However, studies show that environmental stimulation can have different effects on brain structure depending on when it occurs in development (Greenough et al., 1987). For example, animals can be permanently blinded if they are reared in total darkness for 2 weeks right after birth. However, if the deprivation occurs somewhat later in the postnatal period, their visual skills develop normally. To explain such time-dependent results, Greenough et al. (1987) proposed that mammalian brain development involves two types of neural plasticity: experience-expectant and experience-dependent. *Experience-expectant* plasticity exploits regularities in the environment to shape developing neural systems. Appropriate circuits develop if the animal experiences these regularities (e.g., contrast borders, movement, etc.).

The mechanism of change in experience-expectant plasticity appears to be an early overproduction of synapses followed by a pruning of exuberant projections in response to experience. The overproduction of synapses is said to take place in order to compensate for possible problems that arise during proliferation and migration (to make sure that there are enough neurons to form a functional circuitry). The pruning takes place because the neurons must compete for a limited supply of trophic factors (as I described earlier).

The second type of plasticity, *experience-dependent*, is thought to have evolved to allow the animal to form representations of unique features of its environment (e.g., characteristics of its own mother, sources of food and haven, native language properties, etc.). The mechanism of change here is not the elimination of excessive synapses as much as the creation of *new* synapses (Greenough et al., 1987; Quartz & Sejnowski, 1997). Or, more accurately, new learning is probably best conceived of as the *reorganization* of synapses (elimination of some combined with the addition of others).

In sum, then, we can attribute the fact that most of us can see (or hear) normally to the fact that we had appropriate visual (or auditory) experiences when we were young. In contrast, we can attribute the fact that we represent a *particular* sensory experience in a particular region of the cortex to the fact that (1) afferents project to that region and (2) we had the experience. It is in this way that experience can sculpt our brains and create a dynamic type of circuitry.

Nutrition

Numerous experimental studies with animals have shown that malnutrition can have different effects on brain development depending on when it occurs (Winick, 1984). Scientists explain such time-dependent outcomes by arguing that early (i.e., prenatal) malnutrition slows the rate at which cells are proliferated, thereby reducing the total number of neurons and glial cells in an animal's brain. Later malnutrition, in contrast, slows the rate at which the already proliferated cells grow in size or acquire a myelin sheath. Whereas the latter problems can be ameliorated by providing enriched diets to malnourished animals, the former problem of too few cells cannot be corrected in this way. Such findings suggest, then, that prenatal malnutrition would cause more permanent harm to developing human brains than postnatal malnutrition (because proliferation largely occurs during the prenatal months in humans).

This claim is supported by various correlational studies of malnourished and normally fed children around the world (e.g., Streissguth, Barr, Sampson, Darby, & Martin, 1989; Winick, 1984) as well as by a recent quasi-experimental study conducted by Pollitt, Gorman, Engle, Martorell, and Rivera (1993). These researchers gave either a high-protein, high-calorie supplement ("Atole") or a low-protein, lower calorie supplement ("Fresco") to poor Guatemalan pregnant women and their children. Some children received the supplement postnatally, while others received it both prenatally and postnatally. Children were followed longitudinally (i.e., over time) and given various assessments when they were preschoolers and adolescents. At the preschool assessment, Pollitt et al. found that children given the Atole supplement performed significantly better than children given the Fresco supplement, even after controlling for gender, age, and socioeconomic status. However, the findings were largely limited to motor skills. At the adolescent assessment, the Atole supplement was associated with higher cognitive skills, but it explained only 1–5% of the variance in these abilities. Factors such as gender, socioeconomic status, and schooling explained much more of the variance. In line with the findings with animals, however, Pollitt et al. found that children who started supplemental feeding after 24 months showed less benefit than children who received the supplement before and after birth.

Taken together, such studies suggest that nutrition has the potential to affect two important aspects of brain development: proliferation and myelination. Studies have also shown that brain development can be enhanced in most children by making sure that they have adequate levels of protein and fatty acids in their diets (Winick, 1984). For children who have the condition known as phenylketonuria (PKU), however, a high-protein diet could prove disastrous if it is left unchecked. Children with PKU are unable to convert the amino acid *phenylalanine* into the amino acid *tyrosine* (Diamond, Prevor, Callender, & Druin, 1997). As a result, they experience two main problems. First, high levels of phenylalanine in the bloodstream causes progressive brain damage and mental retardation. Second, tyrosine is a precursor to dopamine. Circuits comprised of dopaminergic neurons cannot work properly when the level of dopamine is too low.

Whereas the first problem can be alleviated by having PKU children avoid foods that contain high levels of phenylalanine (a strategy that has been in place for many years), researchers have not yet figured out how to solve the second problem (Diamond et al., 1997). As a result, many PKU children still experience subtle cognitive deficits.

Steroids

The term *steroids* refers to a class of hormones in the body that play a role in a number of functions, including the development of sexual characteristics and stress reactions. Scientists believe that steroids affect brain development for four reasons. First, the brain is one of several organs in the body that contain receptors for estrogens and related substances (e.g., cortisol and other stress hormones). As such, there is reason to think that it would be transformed during prenatal development in the same way that other so-called *steroid target tissues* (e.g., genitalia) are transformed (Kelley, 1993). Also, excessive amounts of stress hormones could promote the death of neurons in certain key areas of the brain (see Chapters 5 and 8). The second reason relates to the consistent patterns of gender differences that have been found in areas such as cognitive skills, psychological disorders, and violent behavior. Many scientists believe that the consistency of these differences argues in favor of inborn structural differences in the brains of men and women (Halpern, 1992).

The third reason derives from various experimental studies of animals. In one line of research, scientists uncovered gender differences in brain structure that are visible to the naked eye (Breedlove, 1994). Other studies have shown that sex hormones can alter the brains and behaviors of animals. For example, female rats exposed to androgens have been found to engage in sexual behaviors that are characteristic of male rats (e.g, mounting).

The fourth reason derives from several recent studies that have compared the brains of three groups: homosexual men (Group 1), heterosexual men (Group 2), and heterosexual women (Group 3). The logic of this comparison is as follows: If sexual attraction to men is brain-based, then the brains of people in Group 1 should look more like the brains of people in Group 3 than like the brains of people in Group 2 (Breedlove, 1994). Researchers recently demonstrated this expected pattern for a region of the hypothalamus that has been implicated in sexual functioning. The region was significantly larger in Group 2 than in either Group 1 or Group 3 (which did not differ).

While the results of all of these studies are certainly intriguing, it cannot be said that they convincingly demonstrate that the human brain is sexually dimorphic. The first problem relates to a high level of inconsistency in the evidence reported by researchers who have used either MRI or postmortem methodologies within human brains. Some have found structural differences that are consistent with the behavioral evidence (e.g., larger spatial areas in men), others report differences that are opposite to what would be predicted (e.g., larger spatial areas in women), and a third group has found no structural differences at all (Beaton, 1997; Breedlove, 1994; Driesen & Raz, 1995; Giedd et al., 1996). The second problem is that human behavior is far more flexible and context-sensitive than animal behavior (Breedlove, 1994; Byrnes & Fox, 1998). As such, there is little reason to think that humans and animals would respond in the same way to some experimental intervention (e.g., an injection of androgens). Third, the brain regions targeted by experimental interventions have not been consistently related to sexual behaviors in either animals or humans. Finally, it is not at all clear why the size of a particular brain region would necessarily relate to behaviors in a meaningful way (Breedlove, 1994; Beaton, 1997).

Thus, even though there is reason to think that steroids could alter the brains of men and women, scientists have found little hard evidence of this transformation. This lack of evidence either means that sexual dimorphisms do not exist or that scientists have been looking in the right places but have been using the wrong metrics). With respect to the latter possibility, note that few researchers have investigated whether steroids alter (1) the distribution of particular types of cells in given regions or (2) patterns of connectivity. Such differences could not be detected with MRI technology (because they have little to do with size or shape), but they could be detected in postmortem studies.

Teratogens

Any foreign substance that causes abnormalities in a developing embryo or fetus is called a *teratogen*. Researchers identify teratogens through retrospective analyses, prospective longitudinal studies, and prospective experimental investigations. Using the retrospective technique, mothers of children who are born with birth defects are interviewed to determine whether they may have ingested something (e.g., alcohol) or been exposed to something (e.g., a virus) that could have altered the course of their child's development in utero. Using the prospective longitudinal technique, pregnant women are interviewed regarding their behaviors during their pregnancy and followed for years after they give birth. Of interest is the association between their exposure to teratogens and the developmental outcomes in their children. Using the prospective experimental technique, pregnant animals are exposed to various dosages of suspected teratogens. Their offspring are then analyzed for the presence of physical or behavioral anomalies.

Scientists consider a substance to be a teratogen only if both of the following are true: (1) a sufficient level of evidence has accumulated from retrospective or prospective studies to show a consistent linkage between the substances and birth defects; and (2) the dosages utilized in prospective experimental studies are not unrealistically high. Many common substances (e.g., caffeine and nicotine) have been found to produce birth defects when given at extremely high and unrealistic dosages, but not when given at more realistic levels. Such substances are generally not considered teratogens by scientists, but they may nevertheless appear on lists of to-be-avoided substances issued by the federal government, or on the warning labels of packages. The government takes a more cautious approach since it often takes time to determine whether a substance really is dangerous. Hence, government officials think it is better to be safe than sorry.

Generally speaking, two types of teratogens have been the subject of numerous investigations: viruses and drugs. Viruses reproduce themselves by invading a host cell (e.g., a neuron), releasing their nucleic acids into the surrounding tissue, and coopting the host cell's metabolic machinery. In mature organisms, this invasion usually results in transient symptoms such as lethargy and fever. In developing organisms, however, a viral infection can have more permanent effects if it occurs when the organism's cells are in the midst of proliferating, migrating, or differentiating. Viruses such as rubella have been linked to a range of birth defects including microencephaly (i.e., a small head and brain). It is not yet clear whether other viruses are also linked to abnormal brain development in the same way, but the key seems to be whether the virus targets particular kinds of tissues. Cold viruses and flu viruses target tissues in the nose and lungs, respectively, and do not apparently target developing embryonic tissue (such as developing neurons).

As for drugs or toxic substances, numerous prospective and retrospective studies have been conducted to determine whether substances such as lead, alcohol, marijuana (cannabis), cocaine, caffeine, nicotine, aspirin, acetaminophen, and antihistamine are teratogens. Maternal exposure to high levels of lead has been found to be associated with higher rates of fetal loss (i.e., spontaneous abortion), but lower levels do not appear to produce large-scale cognitive deficits or physical abnormalities in children (Bellinger & Needleman, 1994). Maternal consumption of alcohol, however, has been consistently linked to a range of cognitive and motor deficits (Barr, Streissguth, Darby, & Sampson, 1990; Streissguth et al., 1989; Streissguth et al., 1994). In heavy drinkers and alcoholics, prenatal exposure to alcohol occasionally leads to a disorder called fetal alcohol syndrome, which has an incidence rate of about three per 1,000 births. As for marijuana, cocaine, caffeine, nicotine, aspirin, acetaminophen, and antihistamine, the collective evidence from prospective and retrospective studies with humans suggests that these substances do not appear to be consistently related to long-term cognitive or motoric deficits (Barr & Streissguth, 1991; Hinds, West, Knight, & Harland, 1996; Streissguth et al., 1994). Experimental studies with animals, however, have found teratogenic effects for all of these substances. In each case, there is evidence that the substance has the potential to interfere with the processes of proliferation, migration, and differentiation. In the final section of this chapter, I shall explore possible reasons why these drugs seem to affect the offspring of animals more than the offspring of humans.

Summary

The preceding discussion focused on five factors that have been found to produce individual differences in brain structure: genes, environmental stimulation, nutrition, steroids, and teratogens. This analysis revealed that two people could develop different brains because they (1) had different genes, (2) had differing levels or types of environmental stimulation, (3) ingested differing levels or types of food, (4) were exposed to differing levels or types of steroids, or (5) were exposed to differing levels or types of teratogens. The evidence as a whole, however, suggests that most of the structural differences that might arise between people would tend to be rather small and subtle. Large-scale differences in brains might only arise when several of these factors work in concert, or when extreme values of the individual factors are involved (e.g., shifting from 46 to 47 chromosomes; reducing diets by 60%; rearing animals in the dark; drinking large quantities of alcohol daily; etc.).

CONCLUSIONS AND CAVEATS

In a certain sense, the present chapter represents a "how to" manual for building a human brain. The standard model of this brain is clearly the default option that is likely to emerge in all but the most adverse environments. The underlying principles behind this high degree of adaptive success appear to be two notions:

1. *Overproduction*: Build more brain cells and synaptic connections than most people will need; if proliferation, migration, differentiation, and synaptogenesis are somehow slowed or altered, there may still be enough cells around to create functional circuits.
2. *Flexibility and plasticity*: Augment genetic instructions with cellular feedback loops; make use of both experience-expectant and experience-dependent learning processes; make use of alternative brain regions if the typical brain region lacks functional circuits (the latter mostly applies to young children).

These two principles combined with physical aspects of the intrauterine environment (e.g., crowding, passive migration, etc.) also mean that individual differences in brain structure will be the norm rather than the exception (even in identical twins). However, in most cases, the differences that emerge in brain structure will tend to be rather subtle. Whether any of these smaller differences are responsible for either individual differences in behavior or phenotypic similarity in twins is currently a matter of controversy.

Moreover, it is important to point out that much of what we know (or, rather, *believe*) about brain development is still tentative and fairly controversial. To a large extent, the lack of certainty is due to the fact that researchers have had to resort to experimental studies with animals to determine the possible role of certain factors in development (e.g., environmental stimulation, hormones, etc.). Interspecies differences clearly cloud the conclusions that can be drawn from such studies (see Chapter 1). Moreover, studies with humans are, by necessity, correlational rather than experimental. Any linkages between background variables (e.g., nutrition) and outcomes (e.g., brain size) could be spurious.

What, then, are the implications of the research on brain development for psychological theory, educational practice, and public policy? We have seen that the adult form of a person's brain is jointly a function of (1) genetic instructions that specify the length of the proliferative phase and the kinds and locations of neurons that are produced; (2) mechanical processes involved in the movement of cells and progressive lengthening of axons; (3) chemical signals between neurons (neurotransmitters that are sent across synapses as well as other signals that help guide axonal projections and inform the differentiation process);

(4) environmental stimulation that causes clusters of neurons to fire together, form synapses with each other, and create functional areas of the cortex (e.g., for vision or math); and (5) other factors that interfere with the normal processes of sculpting (e.g., teratogens and diseases). We have also seen that there is not a one-to-one relationship between genes and the final cytoarchitecture of someone's brain and that the human brain is highly plastic in the sense that it can reorganize itself and overcome obstacles imposed by the environment. However, the ability of the brain to overcome problems varies over time. For example, whereas the effects of prenatal malnutrition on the brain seem to be relatively permanent, the effects of postnatal malnutrition seem to be reversible.

When confronted with these tentative conclusions, a variety of reactions seem possible. Some have used the findings in this chapter and related findings to argue in favor of the constructivist orientation to cognitive development (e.g., Quartz & Sejnowski, 1997). The constructivist orientation lies midway between a *nativist orientation*, which espouses the idea that mental representations of such things as faces, math skills, and grammatical categories exist at birth prior to environmental input, and an *empiricist orientation*, which espouses the idea that the mind is a blank slate at birth that is entirely shaped by subsequent environmental input. Among developmental psychologists, there is an ongoing, vigorous debate between the nativist and the constructivist camps, so presumably the findings can be used to bolster the position of the constructivists. Relatedly, most mathematics and science educators espouse the constructivist philosophy these days (Byrnes, 2001), so these educators may use the findings to their advantage as well. However, there is a large gap between finding support for the metatheoretical belief system of constructivism and finding support for a particular theory or instructional technique that is consistent with this paradigm (e.g., Piaget's theory or the instructional approach advocated by the National Council of Teachers of Mathematics). There are many ways to conceptually and behaviorally implement constructivism (in the same way that there are many ideas, behaviors, and rituals consistent with the religious beliefs of Christianity).

Relatedly, some have used the time-dependent relation between environmental input and brain sculpting to argue in favor of such things as starting foreign language and music instruction in the preschool period (before a presumed critical period is over) rather than later in development. Others, in contrast, have argued that nothing at all can be concluded from the time-dependent effects of the environment because they only apply to cases of extreme deprivation (Bruer, 1998). The present author would tend to agree more with the latter than with the former reaction, but would add that the findings are nevertheless important for the attitudes we take toward children. There is an unfortunate tendency for scientists, educators, and ultimately parents to take a deterministic, pessimistic view of abilities and disabilities. The findings regarding plasticity and environmental input show that children are not destined to particular outcomes due to their genes. In other words, there is much we can do to improve skills in children. The sooner we start, the sooner the sculpting and plasticity can begin. In the same way, the findings show that gender and ethnic differences in abilities may be relatively easy to eliminate and that parental guilt over "giving" their children a malady with a presumed genetic basis (e.g., reading disability, autism, etc.) may be misguided. The stochastic, mechanical quality of brain maturation may be the culprit in many cases (i.e., things just did not go as planned by the genes).

CHAPTER 3

Memory

The science of psychology is all about "carving the mind at its joints" (Kosslyn & Koenig, 1992). That is, psychological theorists decompose the mind into a finite number of abilities (e.g., spatial reasoning, memory, language, etc.), and then decompose each of these abilities into a finite number of components (e.g., mental rotation, location memory, and visual tracking in the case of spatial reasoning). At one time, psychologists primarily pointed to behavioral evidence from experiments to back up their claims that a particular ability contained a specific number of components. Now they often appeal to neuroscientific evidence as well (Kosslyn & Koenig, 1992; Posner & Raichle, 1994). This new tendency to use neuroscientific and behavioral evidence reflects two emergent beliefs in the field: (1) behavioral evidence is often equivocal (i.e., the same evidence can usually be explained by at least two theories); and (2) the dichotomy between psychological science and brain science is increasingly thought to be false (see Chapter 1).

In this chapter and the remaining chapters of this book, my general approach will be to describe current psychological opinion regarding the nature of some entity (e.g., memory) and then to review the neuroscientific evidence that is relevant to this entity. In essence, we shall be considering the extent to which the theoretical "carving" proposed by psychologists is consistent with neuroscientific evidence. After doing so, we shall consider the implications of the analyses for psychological theory and educational practice. To accomplish these goals, then, we need to focus on psychological topics that have direct relevance to education and that have been investigated extensively by psychologists and neuroscientists. Topics that meet just one of these two criteria are not considered in this book. For example, personality has been studied by both psychologists and neuroscientists, but research on personality has little relevance to education. Also, students learn about social studies and science in school, but there are no published neuroscientific studies of these topics (to my knowledge). The topics that meet both criteria include memory, attention, emotion, reading, and math. We shall begin with memory in this chapter and cover attention, emotion, reading, and math in Chapters 4 through 7, respectively.

HUMAN MEMORY AS VIEWED BY PSYCHOLOGISTS

Inasmuch as my primary goal in this book is to consider the relevance of neuroscience for psychology and education, I will present no more than a thumbnail sketch of the psychology of memory here (see Anderson, 1995, or Baddeley, 1999, for more comprehensive accounts). This sketch includes a discussion of the basic components of the human memory system that have been alleged by psychologists, as well the main processes that occur within these components. In essence, we shall be examining memory first from the structural perspective and then from the functional perspective (see Byrnes, 1992, for more on the structuralist and functionalist orientations to theorizing).

Components of the Memory System

The question "How does the human memory system work?" is analogous to the question "How does a car engine work?" The most helpful answer to either question is one that describes the parts of the system (e.g., "The engine consists of a battery, a carburetor, . . . "). The key elements of the human memory system include sensory buffers, rehearsal systems, records, cues, working memory, and permanent memory. Let's examine each of these components in turn.

Sensory Buffers

When people experience something (e.g., go to a party, attend a lecture, read a book, etc.), their sensory detectors (located in their eyes, ears, noses, tongues, and skin) and the perceptual systems corresponding to these detectors (located in their brains) register this stimulation, interpret it, and retain it for a very brief period of time. The visual system, for example, retains (or "echoes") visual patterns for only about 1 second and the auditory system retains speech-like patterns for only about 2–3 seconds (Anderson, 1995). The sensory buffer is useful in that it retains stimulation long enough so that your mind can interpret this stimulation (e.g., "I see a cat"; "I hear music"), but it would not be very good if people could only retain their experiences for 1 second. At the very least, students would retain nothing from lectures and would fail every exam they take! Fortunately, the human memory system includes other components and processes besides sensory buffers.

Rehearsal Systems

If someone told you a phone number and you could not write it down, what would you do? If you are like most people, you would probably say the number over and over to yourself. Each time you do, the number "stays alive" for another 2–3 seconds. If you wanted to remember a visual pattern instead of an auditory pattern (e.g., where some office was located in a building; what something looked like), you would probably revisualize it to yourself over and over. In each case, you are using a particular sensory system as a rehearsal system (Anderson, 1995). Based on the work of Alan Baddeley (e.g., Baddeley, 1999), researchers now call the system for rehearsing verbal information the *phonological loop* and the system for rehearsing visual or spatial information the *visuospatial sketch pad*. Among other things, these two systems were proposed to account for the fact that people cannot perform two tasks that require the same system at the same time (e.g., rehearse two verbal lists). People can, however, perform two tasks that require different systems (e.g., rehearse a verbal list while scanning a computer monitor for a visual signal).

At one time, psychologists thought that the phonological loop had a fixed capacity of between five and nine units (e.g., "the magic number 7"). Thus, if someone has a "span" of, say, seven units and she heard someone call out six letters, she could recall all six of them. However, if this person heard someone call out 12 letters, she would probably fail to remember about five of them. These days, scientists believe that it is not the number of items per se that influences what we recall, it is how many we can *rehearse* before the sensory trace for each item fades that matters. For example, since we can say the one-syllable words "wit, sum, harm, bag, top" in 2 seconds, we could recall all five of these words if they were called out. However, we typically cannot say the multisyllabic words "university, opportunity, expository, participation, auditorium" in 2 seconds, so we would probably only recall about two or three of these words (Baddeley, 1999).

Baddeley likens the process of rehearsal to that of a circus performer spinning plates. Each time we rehearse, we "spin the plate" for that item of information to keep it going. If we have many items (e.g., 12) or items that take a lot of time to "spin" (e.g., five-syllable words), the "plates" for those items will stop before we can "spin" them again. A plate stopping is analogous to a sensory trace fading.

Records

The prominent cognitive psychologist John Anderson uses the term "record" to refer to a mental representation of an item of information that is permanently stored in memory (Anderson, 1995). In Anderson's view, when we say that someone "knows" a lot of things, we are really saying that he or she has many records in his or her memory. Many readers of this book have records for such things as their middle name, the town in which they were born, what the answer to "2 + 2" is, and so on.

Over the years, researchers have learned three important things about records. First, people have records corresponding to four types of knowledge: declarative, procedural, conceptual, and episodic (Anderson, 1995; Byrnes, 1999; Squire, 1987). Your *declarative knowledge,* or "knowing that," is a compilation of all of the facts you know. Very often, declarative knowledge can be stated in the form of propositions. Consequently, some researchers contend that our records corresponding to declarative knowledge are propositional in nature (e.g., Kintsch, 1974). A *proposition* is an assertion that can be either true or false (e.g., "Harrisburg is the capital of Pennsylvania [true]"; "There are three cups in a quart [false]"). Many behavioral studies have suggested that declarative knowledge exists in the form of associative networks. In such networks, there are central notions (e.g., "bird") that are connected associatively to facts people know about the central notion (e.g., "can fly"; "lays eggs"; etc.)

Your *procedural knowledge,* or "knowing how to," is a compilation of all of the skills you know and all the habits you have formed. You probably have records for tying your shoes, performing arithmetic, riding a bike, using a word-processing package, frying an egg, and so forth. Unlike declarative knowledge, in which ideas are interconnected in a network, procedures do not seem to form an associative network among themselves (Anderson, 1993). They do seemed to be associated, however, to cues in the environment (e.g., seeing fractions causes one to retrieve a procedure for adding them).

Your *conceptual knowledge,* or "knowing why," is a form of representation that reflects your understanding of your declarative and procedural knowledge (Byrnes, 1999). If you can give an accurate answer (that makes sense to you) explaining why certain declarative facts are true or why procedures work as they do, you have conceptual knowledge. It is one thing to know facts (e.g., diamonds are hard) and another to know why this fact is true (e.g., diamonds are hard because of the density and arrangement of carbon atoms that comprise them). Similarly, it is one thing to know which procedures to use in a particular instance (e.g., the least common denominator method in the case of adding fractions) and quite another to know why this procedure should be used. At this writing, it is not clear whether conceptual knowledge is also stored as a distinct kind of record or whether it is stored in the form of relations among records.

Your *episodic knowledge* might be called "knowing when and where" because it represents (1) where you were when something happened to you (e.g., a marriage proposal) and (2) when this event took place in your life (e.g., in the summer of 1997). This personalized and historical quality of episodic knowledge is the reason why is it also called *autobiographical memory* (Shimamura, 1995). One important feature of episodic memory is the ability to remember the source of the information in your memory. Obviously, knowing some fact (e.g., that President Clinton's middle name is Jefferson) is different than knowing how you came to know this fact (e.g., reading it in the newspaper, hearing it on TV, being told by a friend, etc.).

The foregoing analysis of record types represents an elaboration of an earlier trichotomy that was proposed by psychologist Endel Tulving in the early 1980s: semantic versus procedural versus episodic (Tulving, 1983). In the earlier account, semantic memory referred to declarative and conceptual knowledge associated with language skills (e.g., reading, writing, comprehending). Procedural and episodic memory referred to the same sorts of things described above. One further kind of knowledge that has been alleged by educational psychologists is *conditional knowledge*, which involves knowing when and where to execute a procedure. However, cognitive psychologists have not advocated this kind of knowledge because the conditions of execution are already built into standard theoretical models of procedural knowledge.

Besides assuming that there are four types of knowledge in memory (declarative, procedural, conceptual, and episodic), the second thing that psychologists have proposed is that records can be stored in two types of *codes*, or formats, visual or verbal (Anderson, 1995; Paivio, 1971). For example, your declarative knowledge that German shepards have pointy ears could be stored as a mental image of what these dogs look like, or stored as the factual proposition "German shepards have pointy ears." Similarly, your procedural knowledge of how to fry an egg might be stored as a nonverbal sequence of imagined actions or as a verbalized set of instructions (e.g., "First, turn on the burner. Next, put butter in the pan . . . "). Of course, advocates of dual coding theory argue that people retain information best when it is encoded in both visual and verbal codes (Paivio, 1971).

Third, psychologists have developed two constructs to explain why people have an easier time remembering some things instead of others: strength and activation level (Anderson, 1995). The *strength* of a record is the degree to which it can be retrieved from memory and made available to consciousness. High-strength records are well-learned facts, procedures, explanations, or personal experiences that come easily to mind when you try to remember them (e.g., your first name; how to tie your shoe). Low-strength records are facts or procedures that you have not learned as well and are difficult to recall (e.g., remembering certain presidents or dates; remembering how to factor an equation). Many studies have shown that the amount of *practice* that you engage in affects the strength of a record. Generally speaking, skills or facts that are practiced regularly attain higher levels of strength than skills or facts that are not practiced to the same degree.

The *activation level* of a record corresponds to its current degree of availability. Making a record sufficiently active to the point that you can think about it is analogous to using a fishing pole to lift a fish close enough to the surface that you can see it. This analogy implies that records need to attain a certain threshold value of activity in order that you have the experience of remembering something.

Records that are in a high state of activation are, then, conscious and available. Records that are in a low state of activation are not quite conscious or available (Anderson, 1995). Readers familiar with word-processing packages know how documents can be retrieved from a floppy diskette or a hard drive. Most packages require an author to highlight the title of a paper and then click on it with a mouse to retrieve it. When the paper comes up on the screen, it has (metaphorically) been made "available" for inspection and revision. Hence, it has been put in a high state of "activation." When it is just sitting there on the diskette, it is in a low state of "activation." The human mind is such that when you metaphorically click on a representation to retrieve a memory (e.g., Who wrote *Death of a Salesman?*), sometimes the memory record comes "up" on your mental "screen" and sometimes it does not. High-strength items come up quickly and right away, low-strength items do not.

Putting strength and activation together, then, we can say that whereas activation level has to do with the current state of a record, strength has to do with its potential to be activated. High-strength records are easier to make highly active (i.e., available to consciousness) than low-strength records. Any knowledge that can be made available to consciousness and that can be verbally described is called *explicit knowledge*. Because explicit knowledge is available to consciousness, people are aware of any changes that happen to it. Unconscious knowledge that cannot be articulated is called *implicit knowledge*. An example is the collection of grammatical rules that people use to process and produce language (see Chapter 6). Because implicit knowledge is not available to consciousness, people are unaware of any changes that occur to it.

Psychologists can, however, test for changes in implicit memory using a variety of techniques. One common approach involves the phenomenon known as *priming*. Priming refers to the increased ability to identify or detect a stimulus as a result of its recent presentation (Squire & Knowlton, 1995). Studies suggest that when a given record is activated, the activation of this record seems to "spread" to other records associated with it. For example, consider the case in which someone has records associated in the following way: the record for "Lincoln" is associated with the records for "president," "the Civil War," and "big expensive car." When he or she hears the word "Lincoln," two things happen. First, the record for "Lincoln" becomes more active than it was. Second, some of the activation of the "Lincoln" record spreads to the other three records. The results of many behavioral studies suggest that activation spreads throughout an associative network of records and becomes weaker the farther it travels along the network.

Prior exposure to a stimulus (e.g., seeing the word "Lincoln") is said to prime the record for that stimulus (i.e., raise its activation level) such that it becomes more easily activated the next time. This facilitation is evident when one uses a two-phase fragment completion task. During the first phase, a list of words is presented (e.g., "Lincoln," "banana," "moose," etc.). During the second phase, word stems are shown (e.g., Li _ _ _ _ _, ba _ _ _ _, etc.) and participants are asked to complete the stems. People are far more likely to complete the stems with words they saw before during the first phase (e.g., complete Li _ _ _ _ _ with Lincoln) than people not exposed to these words What is interesting is that people exposed to the words during the first phase do not remember seeing them. Hence, priming reflects a form of implicit (unconscious) knowledge change (Squire & Knowlton, 1995).

Cues

Cues are things in the environment or items in a rehearsal system that are connected to records. More specifically, cues can cause records to shift from being in a state of low activation to being in a state of higher activation. If the level of activation is high enough, the record becomes available to consciousness. For example, if an individual read the question "Who wrote *Death of a Salesman?*" each of the words in this question (e.g., "death," "salesman") could serve as a cue if it is associated with the record of the author. Or, an additional cue might be the prompt "Arthur _____ wrote *Death of a Salesman.*"

When someone repeats a question to him- or herself, the cues are no longer in the environment, but are now items in a rehearsal system. Using our fishing analogy again, cues are like the rod, the reel, and the bait. When we "cast" cues, they sometimes help us pull up a record and make it highly active. Using our word-processing analogy, perceiving a cue is like clicking on a document to retrieve it.

Working Memory versus Permanent Memory

Having explained the constructs of strength, records, cues, and so on, I am finally in a position to explain the last two parts of the memory system: working memory and permanent memory. Working memory is the term used to refer to any information that is currently available for working on a problem (Anderson, 1995). Thus, items in the sensory buffers or rehearsal systems are in working memory, as are permanent records that are in a highly active state. Working memory is a concept that has generally replaced the notion of short-term memory in contemporary cognitive psychology.

We have already seen how information in sensory buffers can fade within a few seconds. In addition, records that are in a highly active state can easily return to a state of low activation if a person is distracted or stops thinking about the idea. It is for this reason that working memory is considered to be a form of *transient* memory (Anderson, 1995). In contrast, permanent memory pertains to a person's storehouse of records. At one time, psychologists used to call permanent memory "long-term memory" and call working memory "short-term memory" based on several classic models of memory (e.g., Atkinson & Shiffrin, 1968). These models have proven to be somewhat incorrect and misleading, so many cognitive psychologists no longer use the terms associated with them.

Main Processes of the Memory System

Having described the main parts of the memory system, I can now turn to a more dynamic description of the operations or sequence of events that take place within this system of parts. Some of these processes relate to the initial formation of records and some relate to retrieving records from permanent memory. Let's examine these two sets of processes in turn.

Forming Permanent Records

Researchers have examined five main processes related to getting information into permanent memory: attention, encoding, rehearsal, elaboration, and consolidation. The construct of *attention* refers to processes related to such things as orienting, acknowledging the presence of a stimulus, and concentrating. Attention is crucial to memory because information cannot enter the memory system unless it is "attended to" (see Chapter 4 for a complete analysis of attention and its role in learning). *Encoding* is the general term for the process of taking sensory information and transforming it into a permanent record. Said another way, encoding is the process of forming a mental representation of something we experience (Anderson, 1995; Newell & Simon, 1972; Siegler, 1991a). Rather than viewing it as photographic or complete, theorists from a variety of perspectives regard encoding as being *selective* and *interpretive*. Selective means that records only include certain aspects of an experience (in contrast, say, to a videotape that encodes everything). Interpretive means that our orientation toward stimulation determines how we encode it. A good example of this phenomenon is how viewers of a presidential debate often think that their candidate won the debate (both can't be right; they only remember when things went well for their candidate during the debate).

Rehearsal is a process that I already described above when I examined rehearsal systems. It is the process of repeating or "reexperiencing" some stimulation over and over. Thus, repeating a phone number over and over is an example of rehearsal. There is a large body of literature that shows that repetition and practice determine the strength of a record. In fact, researchers recently revealed the existence of the *power law of learning* (Anderson, 1995; Newell & Rosenbloom, 1981) that can be stated as such:

$$\text{Strength} = \text{Practice}^b$$

This is an exponential equation (with an exponent between 0 and 1), which means that learners improve their recall the most during the first few study trials. After that point, they can still increase the strength of a record, but the increases will not be so much. For example, if a student studies the material for a test for 10 straight days, he or she might recall only 40% of the material if tested after the first study day, but 80–90%

of the material if tested after the second study day. Between the third and tenth days, he or she might increase to 90–95%. Note how the increase during the last 8 days of 5% is much less than the 40–50% increase between the first and second days.

The third process related to forming a record, *elaborating*, pertains to the process of "going beyond the information given" and embellishing a raw experience with additional details. For example, if you read the sentence "The boy was crying," you could encode the sentence in a fairly impoverished way or embellish your encoding somewhat. For example, you could ask yourself questions such as "Who is this boy?" and "Why is he crying?" Answering such questions causes the encoding to be embellished with and linked to other ideas.

Some researchers have put the notions of encoding and elaborating together to form the construct of *depth of processing* (Anderson, 1995; Craik & Lockhart, 1972). In this view, any experience can be encoded "shallowly" or "deeply." To get a sense of the difference between shallow and deep processing, imagine that you are in class listening to someone with a very unusual accent. When this person says something like "Einstein may have been dyslexic," you may pay little attention to the meaning of this sentence and focus mostly on the person's strange way of pronouncing the words. If so, you have processed this sentence shallowly. On the other hand, if you try to understand the meaning of the sentence, make inferences, and relate the information to what you already know, you have processed it more deeply. Studies show that students have better retention of material when they process information deeply (e.g., Benton, Glover, Monkowski, & Shaughnessy, 1983; McDaniel, Einstein, Dunay, & Cogg, 1986).

Regardless of whether information is processed shallowly or deeply, most records of our experiences seem to be formed in a gradual way. The gradual nature of the record-forming process is an implicit aspect of the aforementioned power law of learning. But it also is made evident by the phenomenon of *retrograde amnesia* (Squire, 1987). Head trauma or electroconvulsive therapy can cause someone to forget everything that occurred a few weeks to a few years before the trauma or the therapy, but not things that occurred more than a few weeks or years before the trauma or the therapy (e.g., 5–10 years before). These findings suggest that a certain period of time has to elapse before the brain fully *consolidates* memory traces and transforms them into permanent records. Other evidence for consolidation comes from studies of interference effects in which past memories are more likely to cause problems for new learning after these memories have become consolidated than before these memories have become consolidated.

Retrieving Records from Permanent Memory

Creating permanent records by way of attention, encoding, rehearsal, elaboration, or consolidation is not all there is to remembering information. Even after people get information *into* memory, they still have the task of getting it *out*. There are three main ways for people to retrieve information from permanent memory: recall, recognition, and inferential reconstruction. *Recall* is the process involved when people are presented with cues and try to retrieve information associated with the cues (Flavell, Miller, & Miller, 1993). For example, if on a test a student is asked "Who was the third president of the United States?," the cues "third" and "president" could prompt the student to retrieve the name "Thomas Jefferson" from permanent memory. In the same way, a person's face often serves as a cue for his or her name.

Recognition is the process involved when people see, hear, smell, touch, or taste something and then have the feeling that they have encountered this sight, sound, smell, feeling, or taste before. In this case, people are matching a stored representation of something to the real thing in the world (Flavell et al., 1993). For example, a student might have the fact that Thomas Jefferson was the third president of the United States stored as a permanent record. When presented with the item "Jefferson was the third president" on a true–false test, she recognizes this fact as being true. Similarly, people have permanent records for many familiar faces. When they see a person whom they know, they match the person's face to the stored representation and recognize him or her. Unlike recall, in which cues activate something merely associated with records, in recognition, cues directly match records.

The third retrieval process, *inferential reconstruction*, is used when cues cause someone to retrieve only a few fragments of a more complete record. Upon retrieving these fragments, people build up a plausible story around the fragments that seems to be a close approximation to the original record (Anderson, 1995). To get a sense of this, think of an experience that you had as a young child (e.g., getting lost in a store). If you tried to tell what happened to a friend, what would you say? The story you develop would be plausible (what *probably* caused you to get lost), but it may not be exactly what happened.

Forgetting

What happens to our memories as time passes? Why is our memory of some things better than our memory of other things? Answers to these questions center around the notion of forgetting. Based on many years of experimentation, psychologists have proposed three views of forget-ting: *decay theory, interference theory*, and the *loss of retrieval cues* view.

Decay theory is the oldest view of forgetting and one that is quite consistent with the view of the average person on the street (Anderson, 1995). The main premise of this view is that the strength of a record weakens over time if no further practice ensues or if it has not been acti-vated for some time. To get a sense of this notion, let's use the conven-tion that the strength of a record is the probability that it can be recalled. For example, if there is a 40% chance that you will give the right answer to the question "What is the square root of 256?," let's say that the strength of the answer "16" is .40. The decay view suggests that a record that starts out with a strength of 1.0 might ultimately weaken to .80, then to .60, then to .40, and so on with the passage of time.

Research has shown that, indeed, the passage of time does seem to affect the retrievability of a record in a strikingly regular way. Across many different types of memories (e.g., for nonsense syllables, TV shows, factual sentences, etc.), studies show that most of what you for-get is lost very early in the game. You continue to forget additional in-formation after this point, but the rate of loss slows. This general trend has been called the *power law of forgetting* (Anderson, 1995). For ex-ample, one study showed that people remember 80% of canceled TV shows 1 year after they are canceled. Between the first and the eighth year after cancellation, retention drops somewhat quickly from 80% to about 58% (a 22% loss). Between the eighth and the fifteenth year, however, retention drops only 3% further (from 58% down to 55%) (Squire, 1989).

So the passage of time is an important factor in retrievability. But it has also been found that the amount of practice affects forgetting as well. As I noted earlier, practice affects the initial strength of a record. Research has shown that, at any point in time, people who have engaged in more practice show a greater likelihood of retrieving a memory than people who have not practiced as much. Nevertheless, even people who practice a lot show the exact same *rate* of forgetting as people who prac-tice less (Anderson, 1995). So, for example, if Person *A* practiced some-thing 50 times, she might show a drop from 80% correct to 50% right away (a 30% drop) and then level off to 45% over time (a 5% drop). If Person *B* practiced something 100 times, he might go from 100% cor-rect down to 70% (a 30% drop) and level off at 65% (a 5% drop). Thus, the rate of loss is the same, but at each point Person *B* would re-call more than Person *A*. Anderson (1995) has put the two factors of time and practice together in the same schematic function:

$$\text{Strength} = A \times \text{Practice}^{b} \times \text{Delay}^{-c}$$

The A is simply some constant. Notice that the superscript for practice is positive (meaning that more practice yields greater strength) and the superscript for delay is negative (meaning strength is less as time passes). By multiplying these factors together, we see that practice can ameliorate some of the effects of time.

What is interesting about the power law of forgetting is that our minds seem to be naturally equipped to retain only those events that repeat on a regular basis. That is, our minds seem to be saying "This event keeps happening, so I better remember it; that event has not happened for some time and did not repeat very much when it did—I don't need to remember it." Researchers have found that there is a strong correlation between the frequency with which things occur in the environment (e.g., the number of times a person's name is mentioned on a daily basis in the newspaper) and the likelihood that people can recall this information (Anderson & Schooler, 1991).

Although time and practice do seem to affect how much we forget, these factors are not the whole story. Sometimes an *interference* relation can develop between information already in memory and information that we are just learning. When newly learned information causes students to have trouble remembering old information, "retroactive" interference is occurring. For example, first and second graders spend a lot of time learning the fact that "3 + 4 = 7." When they learn a new multiplication fact in third grade such as "3 × 4 = 12," the new associative relation between "3," "4," and "12" may interfere with the old associative relation between "3," "4," and "7." Thus, when asked, "What is 3 + 4?," they may answer "12." In this case, the "3" and the "4" are acting as retrieval cues that activate the record for "12" instead of the record for "7." To overcome this problem, students need to form a four-way association between "3," "4," "×," and "12," as well as between "3," "4," "+," and "7."

When old information interferes with retention of new information, "proactive" interference is occurring. An example of proactive interference would be the case of a third grader responding "7" when asked "What is 3 × 4?" Another example would be an adult giving an old phone number when asked for his or her new number. In the latter case, the phrase "phone number" is a retrieval cue that is associated with both numbers, but is associated more strongly with the old number than it is with the new number.

At this point it is worth noting that from the standpoint of both decay theory and interference theory, forgetting is not seen as information "evaporating" out of memory. Instead, both views consider forgetting to be a problem of pulling up information that is still there (i.e., activating a record to a high enough level). Where these views differ is in how they explain *why* a record fails to attain a high enough level of activation.

The third explanation of forgetting involves the weakening of associations among retrieval cues and records (Anderson, 1995; Tulving & Psotka, 1971). Sometimes we see a face out of context and have the curious feeling that we know that person. For example, I might see one of my students at the grocery store. When this student is currently in one of my classes, the student's face is still strongly associated with the classroom context and other things such as his or her name. So, I can ask myself, "Is this one of my students?," imagine my classes, and then "see" the student in one class. These cues together help me then to recall the student's name. However, when I see a student from many years ago, the associations among the face, classroom, names, and so forth weaken to the point that I am not even sure that the familiar face is a former student!

The readers of this book have also probably had the experience of trying to remember something in the middle of taking a test. Sometimes contextual cues such as the place you wrote something in your notes can serve as a retrieval cue to help you remember. Although such contextual cues may help you right after studying, they will lose their association to information over time. When asked the same test question many months later, you probably will be unable to recall the information.

Memory Strategies and Metamemory

At this point, readers should have a good sense of the nature of retention and forgetting. In what follows, we will examine some things that students can do to help themselves remember information better. As we shall see, certain memory strategies work because they exploit the properties of memory that were described earlier. Although students use many different strategies, we shall briefly focus on five that have received the most attention from researchers: rehearsal, organization, elaboration, the method of loci, and the keyword method. After describing the five strategies, I shall explore a component of the memory system that plays an important role in whether or not we use strategies: metamemory.

As I mentioned earlier, *rehearsal* is the strategy of repeating information over and over. Why does repetition work? It seems that our minds are naturally sensitive to the statistical properties of the environment. We are built to remember things that we are likely to encounter again and to forget rare events. Many studies have confirmed the important role of repetition (Anderson, 1995).

Organization is the strategy of arranging to-be-remembered material into subgroups and hierarchies of subgroups. For example, if asked to study the following 15 items—carrot, truck, cake, broccoli, bike, bus, ice cream, peas, train, potato, candy, pudding, plane, squash, soda—you might form them into three groups (i.e., veggies, vehicles, and sweet stuff) instead of studying them individually. That way, you can use the labels of these groups as retrieval cues when you are later asked to remember the items on the list (e.g., "OK, there were five veggies . . . "). Studies have shown that when students create their *own* organization, they often demonstrate better recall than when teachers or researchers give them an organization. This finding has been called the *generation effect* (McDaniel, Waddill, & Einstein, 1988). Organization also helps recall because the process of forming the categories often promotes the construction of elaborated representations of the material.

The third strategy, *elaboration,* is the practice of imposing meaning of any kind on material. We just learned that organization is one form of elaboration, but the prototypical example of elaboration comes from experiments involving paired-associates learning. When people are presented with pairs of words such as cat–ribbon and elephant–pin, they tend to form mental images that link one term to another. For example, they might imagine the cat wearing the ribbon or the elephant getting stuck by the pin. Either way, the use of such interactive imagery has been found to be a highly effective way to learn the pairs (Weinstein & Mayer, 1986).

There are two reasons why elaboration works as a strategy. First, as the name implies, elaboration involves the creation of an elaborative encoding of the material. This elaboration is especially helpful when it involves linking verbal material to imagery. Second, when students are free to make up their own images, the generation effect comes into play (moreover, the image serves as an additional retrieval cue for either word).

The fourth strategy, the *method of loci,* involves linking up a familiar routine with a series of items that you are trying to learn. Typically, researchers ask students to take a list of facts and then to mentally "attach" each fact to landmarks along a route that is very familiar to them. For example, students who have driven to college the same way every day for 4 years are highly familiar with this route and can imagine it easily. When given a list of, say, 20 facts to learn for a test, students can divide their routes into 20 landmarks along the way (e.g., their neighbor's house, the grocery store on the corner, the church on the next corner, etc.). Then, they can imagine each fact plastered on each of the land-marks. When test time comes, they merely think about their route and the material can be "read" off this image.

The method of loci works for a variety of reasons. Once again, we have elaborative encoding of the material. In addition, students are exploiting their natural capacity to remember visual material better than verbal material and they are linking up the verbal with the visual as suggested by dual coding theory (Paivio, 1971). Third, in selecting which landmarks to use, the generation effect is operative again. Fourth, the fixed sequence of events imposes an organization on material that may not have an organization. Fifth, each landmark or its label can serve as an additional retrieval cue.

The final strategy, the *keyword method*, is particularly useful for learning verbal material such as new vocabulary words (Pressley, Levin, & Delaney, 1982). In this approach, a student takes a new word and finds a portion of it that may be a familiar-sounding, easy-to-imagine term within the word. For example, with the word *caterwaul* a student might identify both "cat" and "wall" (notice that homonyms can be used). When the student learns that *caterwaul* means a noisy fight, he or she can imagine two cats fighting and screeching on a wall. Or, with the Spanish word *carta* (meaning "letter"), a student could see the term "cart" and imagine a letter being transported in a shopping cart. This approach appears to be effective because it involves the generation effect, use of imagery, and cues that are tied to well-learned ideas.

Of the five strategies described above, which do you think would be most effective for studying for a test? Do you use any of these strategies? Would you be more likely to use a particular strategy (e.g., organization) for an essay test than for a multiple-choice test? The answers that you give to these questions derive from your metamemory. The term *metamemory* refers to a person's knowledge and beliefs about how his or her memory works (Flavell, Miller, & Miller, 1993). Perhaps the two most important aspects of metamemory concern: (1) the recognition that your memory is not flawless and (2) knowledge of what strategies to use in particular circumstances. Metamemory has also been extended to such things as the feeling-of-knowing that people get when they retrieve the answer to a question and estimate the likelihood that they are right (Shimamura, 1995).

Strategies are things that you do to avoid forgetting something important. But in order to use a strategy, you have to first recognize that there is some likelihood that you might forget something unless you engage in a strategy. At an even more basic level, strategy users are people who recognize that they sometimes forget. In contrast to good rememberers who know when they are likely to forget something (e.g., they say "I'd better write that down"), poor rememberers think that they never forget. As a consequence, poor remembers never use strategies and forget a great deal (though they do not recognize this!).

Besides recognizing that they forget, good rememberers know which strategies are effective for them and which are not. For example, a good student might discover that the method of loci never works for her but the keyword method does. Upon learning this, she stops using the method of loci. Similarly, a good student might also recognize that rehearsal works well for learning lists of facts, but that various imagery techniques work better for remembering textbook material. Thus, this student would flexibly shift from rehearsal to imagery as his tasks changed from learning lists to reading textbooks.

Summary

In the preceding section, the main parts and processes of the human memory system were described. The parts included such things as records, cues, working memory, and permanent memory. The processes included such things as encoding, retrieval, strategies, and metamemory. As I noted earlier, this account was proposed by psychologists to explain behavioral evidence from a large number of laboratory experiments. In the next section, we shall examine the extent to which the foregoing psychological account squares with evidence that has accumulated from neuroscientific studies.

HUMAN MEMORY AS VIEWED BY NEUROSCIENTISTS

Before one can adequately assess the compatibility of the neuroscientific and psychological views of memory, it is first necessary to consider the ways in which neuroscientific evidence *could be* consistent with (or inconsistent with) a given psychological theory. As I noted earlier, theories carve up the mind into a specific number of components. In a typical psychological experiment, theory-driven hypotheses usually take the form, "If theory X is right that capacity Y consists of components A, B, and C, then people should behave in the following way when presented with the experimental stimuli. . . . " Theory X gains support to the extent that people behave in the predicted way (e.g., remember some items but not others). But what form should hypotheses take when a given capacity is studied from a neuroscientific perspective?

It turns out that the link between psychological theory and neuroscientific evidence is a little less direct. Cognitive neuroscientists generally begin with the assumption that a good way to proceed is to find brain areas that correspond to the components specified in the theory (Kosslyn & Koenig, 1992; Posner & Raichle, 1994). If such brain areas exist, then at least three kinds of methodologies can be used to support the theory: (1) case studies of brain-injured individuals, (2) surgical studies with animals, and (3) neuroimaging techniques (see Chapter 1). Hypotheses for the first two methodologies would take the form, "If theory X is right that capacity Y consists of components A, B, and C, then patients (or animals) with lesions in brain areas J, K, and L should behave in the following way when presented with the experimental stimuli. . . . " In contrast, hypotheses for the neuroimaging approach would take the form, "If theory X is right that capacity Y consists of components A, B, and C, then brain areas J, K, and L should show heightened activity when participants are presented with the experimental stimuli." Theories gain support to the extent that (1) brain-injured individuals or surgically altered animals behave in the manner specified or (2) the brain areas predicted to be active are, in fact, active.

But it is important to note that theory testing is only one of several ways to use neuroscientific evidence in the service of psychological theory. Another fairly common approach (which might be called the *diagnostic approach*) is to use widely accepted theories as "road maps" to help identify the possible deficits of brain-injured individuals (Byrnes & Fox, 1998). Here, researchers compare the performance of brain-injured and control individuals on a series of standard memory tasks. If patients can only perform some of the tasks that can be performed by control subjects, researchers use this difference to speculate about the skills that the patients seem to lack. In so doing, however, they implicitly assume that the widely accepted theories are correct (i.e., they are not really testing the theory as much as using it "as is").

In recent years, researchers have examined the neuroscientific evidence that has accumulated from a large number of diagnostic and theory-testing studies in order to identify the brain structures that seem to be associated with the component parts and processes of the human memory system. Some of the components that have been investigated to date include (1) records, (2) working memory, (3) long-term storage, (4) recall and recognition, (5) interference, and (6) metamemory.

Records

As predicted by the psychological account of records (see above), PET scan studies (e.g., Posner et al., 1988) have shown that deceptively simple stimuli (e.g., single words) are often represented in a number of different codes (e.g., visual, phonological, articulatory, and semantic). To demonstrate the phenomenon of multiple codes, Posner et al. (1988) employed the subtraction technique in which subjects first fixate on a point and then either look at a word that is presented visually or listen to one that is presented orally. Then the researcher subtracts (pixel by pixel) the computed image for the fixation point from the computed image for the other conditions. The brightness of each pixel corresponds to the degree of blood flow to that area. Whereas visually presented words activate five regions of the occipital lobe (over and above the activation caused by fixating on the point), auditory presentation activates both the primary auditory cortex (superior regions of the temporal lobes) and a region of the left temporoparietal cortex that has been related to language processing. These same occipital and temporal areas are also argued to be the storage sites for visual and auditory encodings, respectively (Squire, 1987; Kosslyn & Koenig, 1992).

In addition to asking subjects to simply look at words, Posner et al. (1988) also asked them to pronounce and define the words. By subtracting the activation associated with pronouncing the words from that associated with defining them, Posner et al. were able to identify two regions that seem to be uniquely associated with semantic processing. One of the regions is located in the anterior left frontal lobe and is associated with language fluency (McCarthy & Warrington, 1990). The other region is located in the medial frontal lobe, in an area that seems to support "attention for action" (i.e., attending in order to respond to the enviroment). Lesions of this area have sometimes produced akinetic mutism (Posner et al., 1988). The latter is a temporary disorder of aimless lethargy that sometimes follows injury to the frontal lobes.

Other studies using PET technology have led to similar results. For example, Martin, Wiggs, Ungerleider, and Haxby (1996) found that subjects naming pictures of animals activates regions of the brain that are not active when subjects name pictures of tools (and vice versa). Interestingly, naming tools activates the same area that is active when subjects are asked to imagine hand movements. Similarly, Martin, Haxby, Lalonde, Wiggs, and Ungerleider (1995) found that object naming, color naming, and action word naming all activate unique areas of the cortex. Thus, the records for different kinds of knowledge (e.g., the color of something, the actions associated with it, etc.) are stored in different regions of the cortex.

Recent studies of brain-injured individuals have corroborated these findings. For example, Tranel et al. (1997) revealed an association between the location of lesions and problems identifying persons, animals, and tools. Lesions in the right temporal polar region were most often associated with defective recognition of persons. In contrast, defective recognition of tools was associated with maximal lesion overlap in the left occipital–temporal–parietal junction of the left hemisphere, and defective recognition of animals was associated with lesions in the right mesial occipital/ventral temporal region and left mesial occipital region.

As for different types of memory, Squire and Knowlton (1995) based the taxonomy shown in Figure 3.1 on findings regarding double dissociations in brain-injured patients (see Chapter 1 or the Glossary for a definition of double dissociation). As can be seen, these authors argue that structures in the medial temporal lobe (i.e., the hippocampus, entorhinal cortex, parahippocampal cortex, and perirhinal cortex) and the diencephalon (e.g., the thalamus) seem to be important for declarative (explicit) memory. As for nondeclarative (implicit) memory, double dissociation studies suggest that the striatum is a particularly important structure for the acquisition of sensorimotor skills and habits. The striatum is one of several subcortical structures that collectively comprise the *basal ganglia* (located near structures such as the thalamus and amygdala). Priming, another form of nondeclarative memory, is said to take place between neural circuits located in the cortex itself. Classically conditioned emotional reactions are said to be mediated by the amygdala, while classically conditioned muscular reactions are said to be mediated by the cerebellum. The final kind of nondeclarative memory,

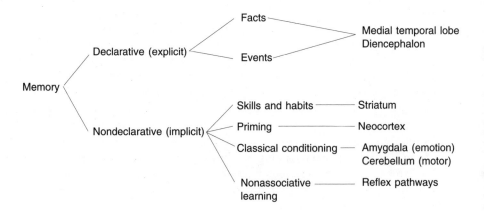

FIGURE 3.1. Brain structures associated with different kinds of memory. After Squire and Knowlton (1995).

nonassociative learning, is said to be linked to reflex pathways located mainly in the spinal cord.

To recap, then, we have seen that there is neuroscientific evidence consistent with the idea that there are five kinds of memory: explicit, implicit, semantic, conceptual, and procedural. To this list, one can add findings from recent PET studies that have investigated episodic memory. Here, frontal cortical regions have been found to be more active when subjects think about their own personal experience than when they think about historical news events (i.e., happenings they know about but did not themselves participate in). The latter activity seems to activate more posterior regions of the cortex (Tulving et al., 1994). Subjects who are asked to listen to previously presented versus novel sentences have PET scans that reveal two bandlike strips of increased activity in the frontal lobes (one in the right dorsolateral frontal cortex and the other in the anterior portion of Brodmann Area 6) and two others in regions of the parietal lobes (Tulving et al., 1994). Tulving et al. argued that these frontal and parietal areas subserve the conscious recollection of previously experienced events (i.e., episodic memory). In a related way, recent evidence from brain-damaged individuals also supports the claim that episodic memory is associated with regions in the frontal lobes (Squire & Knowlton, 1995).

Working Memory

Two experimental paradigms have been used to determine the location of brain regions associated with working memory. In the first, the brains of experimental animals (e.g., monkeys) are lesioned in specific areas. Then the animals are given tasks to perform that place greater or lesser demands on their working memory. In one task, for example, the animal watches which an experimenter places a bit of food into one of two wells in front of it. Then the experimenter draws a shade that hides the wells from the animal for a few seconds, requiring the animal to keep in mind the location of the food. Finally, the shade is drawn back and the animal is allowed to retrieve the food. Studies such as these suggest that there is a working memory network that includes the prefrontal cortex (in the frontal lobes) and several areas to which this cortex is connected (especially the parietal cortex, hippocampus, and thalamus). The primary function of neurons in the prefrontal cortex is to excite or inhibit activity in other parts of the brain (Goldman-Rakic, 1992). It is possible, therefore, that the prefrontal area may serve as a coordinator of activity in situations requiring working memory.

In the second line of research, scientists record the brain activity of humans as they engage in tasks that require different kinds of working memory. These studies (e.g., Smith, Jonides, & Koeppe, 1996) suggest that verbal working memory tasks excite Brodmann Area 40 of the left parietal lobe and three areas in the left frontal lobe: Broca's area (Area 44), the inferior aspect of the premotor area (Area 6), and the superior aspect of the supplementary motor area (Area 6). Spatial tasks, in contrast, excite three regions in the right hemisphere: the ventrolateral frontal cortex (Area 47), Area 19 of the occipital lobe, and Area 40 in the parietal cortex.

Thus, both lines of evidence converge on the idea of a network of working memory areas located mainly in the frontal lobes and parietal lobes of each hemisphere (though the left–right dissociation for verbal and spatial memory has obviously only been found for the one species that has spoken language: humans). The frontal and parietal areas are known to have reciprocal connections with each other, suggesting that activity in one area can instigate activity in the other.

One further point relates to the fact that the prefrontal cortex is rich in neurons that express dopamine (Goldman-Rakic, 1992). In Chapter 2, we saw that children who have the disorder PKU often have a deficiency of dopamine in their brains. Diamond et al. (1997) put these two facts together to design an experiment in which they demonstrated a difference in working memory ability between children with PKU and controls.

Long-Term Storage

Earlier we learned that there is behavioral evidence in support of the theoretical distinction between working memory and permanent memory. It turns out that there is neuroscientific evidence in support of this distinction as well. For example, the literature on brain injuries is replete with suggestions of double dissociations between working memory and long-term storage. Patients with frontal lobe damage generally do not show a deficit in the learning of new material, but they do show a deficit in working memory (Shimamura, 1995; Squire & Knowlton, 1995). In contrast, patients with damage to medial temporal areas (e.g., the hippocampus) and diencephalic structures (e.g., the thalamus) have severe problems in learning new information, but they do not have trouble maintaining information in working memory (Squire, 1987).

The medial temporal areas are thought to be important for the consolidation of permanent records, but it is not yet clear how these structures facilitate consolidation. One recent suggestion is that the hippocampus may temporarily bind together disparate cortical sites associated with a memory (e.g., what an object looks like, what its name is, etc.) until the permanent cortico–cortico connections that constitute the record are established (Squire & Alvarez, 1998). As this account and related accounts suggest, *learning* (i.e., forming a permanent record of declarative, conceptual, procedural, and episodic knowledge) *involves the establishment of relatively permanent synaptic connections among neurons.*

Recall and Recognition

As noted earlier, healthy individuals can greatly increase their chances of recalling something if they use strategies during both the storage and the retrieval phases of memory. For example, they might group items into categories during the storage phase (e.g., plants, animals, and vehicles), and then later use the labels of these categories as self-generated cues during the retrieval phase (e.g., "OK, there were plants, animals, and vehicles; the plants were. . . . "). But the key term here is *healthy*, because strategy use would not be expected to enhance recall performance in individuals who have lesions in brain areas associated with record-formation and consolidation processes (e.g., medial temporal and diencephalic structures; see above).

More generally, the neuroscientific perspective combined with the psychological perspective helps us to understand each of the following four possibilities: (1) strategy use leads to enhanced memory, (2) strategy use does not lead to enhanced memory, (3) enhanced memory occurs even though strategies are not used, and (4) strategies are not used and memory is not enhanced. The first possibility applies to healthy individuals and individuals who have brain injuries in areas that are not specifically associated with record-formation or consolidation processes. For example, frontal lobe patients tend not to use strategies, but their memory performance improves when they are asked to do so (Shimamura, 1995). The second possibility applies to adults who have lesions in medial temporal and diencephalic structures, children and adults with learning disabilities, and preschool children (Flavell, Miller, & Miller, 1993; Squire & Knowlton, 1995; Stanovich, 1988a). In all these groups, strategy use often fails to lead to enhanced performance. The third possibility applies to situations involving incidental memory enhancements, implicit memory (e.g., priming), and enhancement due to emotional arousal (see Chapter 6). The fourth possibility applies to all individuals, regardless of their health status. Collectively, these four possibilities show how neuroscientific evidence can qualify or even explain the outcomes of psychological experiments on recall.

As for recognition, Mishkin and Murray (1998) recently constructed the schematic diagram in Figure 3.2 as a means of summarizing what is currently believed about the neurobiological basis of this form of memory. Higher order sensory areas in the cortex (e.g., Area V1 in the occipital lobes in the case of vision) interpret input from the sensory modalities (e.g., the eyes). This information is passed to a circuit comprised by two cortices in the medial temporal region (i.e., the perirhinal and entorhinal cortex), and also to the medial thalamus, basal forebrain, and orbital region of the frontal lobes. Disruptions in recognition memory have been found when any of these structures are damaged, though damage to the medial temporal structures seems to be particularly important.

Interference

Proactive interference occurs when previously learned information (e.g., an old phone number) makes it hard to remember new information (e.g., a new phone number). Healthy individuals can overcome proactive interference in two ways. First, they can engage in more practice to increase the strength of the record associated with the new information. Second, they can engage in active inhibition of the old information.

Studies show that frontal lobe patients are particularly susceptible to proactive interference (Shimamura, 1995). This finding makes sense given the fact that the frontal lobes make both excitatory and inhibitory connections with other regions of the cortex (Goldman-Rakic, 1992).

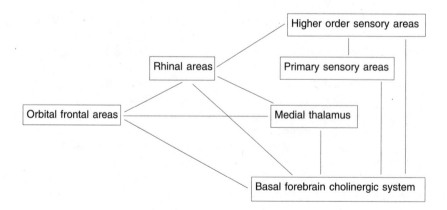

FIGURE 3.2. Schematic of brain areas associated with recognition memory. After Mishkin and Murray (1998).

Metamemory

The frontal lobes have also been implicated in a handful of studies that examined the neuroscientific basis of metamemory. Damage to the frontal lobes has been found to affect (1) knowledge estimation skills, (2) the tip-of-the-tongue phenomenon, (3) the "feeling of knowing," (4) source memory, and (5) recognizing the need to use memory strategies (Shimamura, 1995).

Summary

A useful way to summarize the neuroscientific evidence discussed above is to group together all skills that are associated with particular regions of the brain. The frontal lobes, for example, have been implicated in word finding, episodic memory, working memory, interference, strategies, and metamemory. The temporal lobes, in contrast, are associated with the processing and storage of auditory representations, declarative (explicit) memory, consolidation, recall, recognition, and semantic memory. As for the parietal and occipital lobes, studies suggest that whereas the former is associated with working memory and episodic memory, the latter is associated with the processing and storage of visual representations, spatial working memory, and the recognition of animals. The subcortical structures associated with memory include the basal forebrain (recognition), striatum (sensorimotor skills and habits), amygdala (classically conditioned emotional reactions), and cerebellum (classically conditioned motor responses).

CONCLUSIONS AND CAVEATS

Two conclusions seem appropriate, given the arguments presented so far: (1) human memory is multifaceted and widely distributed across many regions of the brain; (2) the psychological and neuroscientific perspectives on memory appear to be largely consistent with each other. Both of these conclusions, if corroborated in additional, well-controlled experiments, could have important implications for the field of psychology and related disciplines (e.g., education). In what follows, several of these implications are drawn out for illustrative purposes.

The first implication for the field derives from the central role played by human memory in various cognitive abilities including reading, writing, speaking, problem solving, object permanence, and spatial reasoning (Baddeley, 1999; Byrnes, 2001; Goldman-Rakic, 1992). If memory is, in fact, multifaceted and distributed, one could reasonably assume that memory-dependent skills are also multifaceted and distributed. As we shall see in subsequent chapters, this expectation is repeatedly borne out.

The second implication pertains to the notion of parsimony. For most of this century, psychologists have regularly argued that preference should always be given to the more parsimonious of two competing theoretical explanations. This notion is so entrenched that it sometimes causes scholars to reject proposals that contain a high degree of common sense (e.g., stimuli encoded in both verbal and spatial formats are easier to recall than stimuli encoded in just the verbal format). The model of memory that is presented in this chapter is far from parsimonious, but it is more accurate than simpler models that were the standard only 30 years ago (e.g., Atkinson & Shiffrin, 1968). At the very least, this complexity means that we have to start responding to questions such as "Does memory change with age?" by asking our own follow-up questions such as "Which aspect of memory do you mean?"

The third and final implication pertains to the relevance of the psychological and neuroscientific research on memory to instructional practice. Much has been made in the popular press about the idea that "learning is in the synapses." Some authors of practitioner-oriented texts and articles, for example, have gone so far as to suggest that (1) things are learned better if more synapses are formed during a lesson and (2) divergent thinking promotes a wider array of synaptic connections. Unfortunately, however, the synaptic basis of learning is largely irrelevant to modes of instruction. In other words, we have no reason to think that one instructional technique is more likely to promote an optimal form of synaptogenesis than another (especially since there is not a one-to-one correspondence between a given experience and a set of neural connections).

What one can do is base one's instructional decisions on the *psychological* model of learning and memory that is highly consistent with both behavioral *and* neuroscientific evidence. The description of memory provided in the first part of this chapter is just such a model. It suggests that instruction is likely to succeed (i.e., create semipermanent records) if it (1) involves practice and (2) helps children to create elaborated, multicode representations. Teachers should evaluate particular curricular packages in these terms.

CHAPTER 4

Attention

Over 100 years ago, the eminent U.S. psychologist William James wrote the following about attention: "Everyone knows what attention is. It is the taking possession by the mind, in clear and vivid form, of one out of what seem several simultaneously possible objects or trains of thought. Focalization, concentration, [and] consciousness are its essence. It implies withdrawal from some things in order to deal effectively with others . . . " (James, 1890). This cogent description highlights several important aspects of attention that have withstood the test of time.

First, consider James's claim that everyone knows what attention is. It seems that most people can readily identify situations in which they were not paying attention to something, as well as other situations in which they were paying a great deal of attention. In other words, attention has a certain phenomenology, or "feel," to it (i.e., we know what it feels like to pay attention). Another apparent reason for attention's familiarity is the fact that there are many natural language expressions for attention-related experiences that regularly appear in the conversations of scientists and nonscientists alike (e.g., "paying attention," "spacing out," "daydreaming," "concentrating," etc.).

Second, there is the notion that attention is *selective* rather than all-inclusive. Much like the lens of a camera, our minds seem to focus clearly on some things in a situation to the exclusion of others. The unattended objects seem to fade into the background or are missed entirely. Third, there is the idea that attention can be applied in *varying degrees* to some object. Concentrating on an object intensely does not seem to be the same thing as merely looking at it.

Over the years, scientists have attempted to elaborate on William James's original account from both psychological and neuroscientific perspectives. My goal in the present chapter is to summarize these elaborations. Using the same organizational scheme that I utilized in Chapter 3, I present the psychological perspective first and the neuroscientific perspective second. In the final section, I address the instructional implications of recent attempts to integrate the psychological and neuroscientific views of attention.

Before proceeding, however, I must reintroduce the criteria by which the topics in this book were selected (including attention). Topics were included if (1) they have been studied by both psychologists and neuroscientists, and (2) they are directly relevant to the process of education. The former criteria allows one to compare the degree of overlap between the psychological and the neuroscientific perspectives on a particular topic, and also keeps this book from becoming a treatise on all aspects of neuroanatomy (most of which are far removed from the fields of psychology and education). The second criteria limits the topics to those that have relevance to the classroom. Some topics have been intensively studied by psychologists but have been given scant attention by neuroscientists (e.g., nonappetitive aspects of motivation such as goals and self-efficacy; scientific thinking). Other topics have been studied by both psychologists and neuroscientists but have little direct relevance to classroom practice (e.g., personality traits). The topic of attention meets both selection criteria. Apart from being intensively studied by psychologists and neuroscientists for quite some time, attention can also be considered a "gateway to learning." All the major theorists in the area of learning agree that information in a lesson cannot be learned if children are not paying attention. Moreover, anyone who has spent time in the classroom or coached children below the age of 10 knows how often children are off-task and how easily they can be distracted. Why do children seem to attend better with age? Does it have anything to do with brain maturation? Further, some of the pioneers in the area of the linkage between brain science and educational practice have argued that attention may be the key process by which neuroscience and education interface (as described below).

PSYCHOLOGICAL PERSPECTIVES ON ATTENTION

Over the years, psychologists have explained the construct of attention in a variety of ways. In the present chapter, I will examine seven of these viewpoints in turn: (1) information-processing theory, (2) the life-span perspective, (3) Vygotsky's theory, (4) emergent motivation theory, (5) "flashbulb" memories, (6) the educational perspective, and (7) the clinical perspective.

The Information-Processing View

Since the late 1950s, psychological descriptions of attention have been largely based on the principles and practices of information-processing (IP) theory. IP theorists (e.g., Atkinson & Schiffrin, 1968; Broadbent, 1958; Newell & Simon, 1972) argue that the human mind is analogous to a computer in two important ways: (1) both manipulate and process symbols and (2) both carry out operations using a limited amount of processing capacity (e.g., RAM in the case of a computer and working memory in the case of a human mind). The constraints on processing capacity affect the amount of information that can be attended to at one time, and also the manner in which information can flow within the system. So, for example, IP theory suggests that a person would not remember everything about a situation. Instead, he or she would encode only the fraction of the situation that could fit within the capacity of what was then called the short-term memory store (and is now called working memory; see Chapter 3). Similarly, a person could not simultaneously process two information streams that required the same operating system. The latter type of constraint is exemplified by the so-called cocktail party phenomenon in which we can listen to and comprehend the utterances of only one person at a time. When many people talk at once, most of us say things like "Whoa, slow down, one at a time!"

Several different models of attentional processes have been proposed by IP theorists over the years. In Broadbent's (1958) early model, attention was viewed as a set of channels that could carry information. A key assumption of this model was that information could only flow along one channel at a time. This limitation implied that if there were information in both an "open" and a "blocked" channel, only the information in the open channel would be processed and retained. Some studies in the 1960s, however, showed that a certain amount of the unattended to information does seem to get processed (Posner, 1995). As a result, subsequent models shifted away from Broadbent's all-or-none approach to ones that assumed that stimulation from several different channels could simultaneously compete for the same limited amount of attentional resources (Glover, Ronning, & Bruning, 1990). Later proposals also fused attentional constructs with the idea of working memory. In the latter accounts, researchers argued that information is lost not because it fails to get into sensory registers or working memory (as

Broadbent claimed). Rather, information gets lost because there are only so many things in working memory that can be attended to before the sensory traces of each bit of information fades (see Chapter 3).

In addition to suggesting that people could not encode everything in a situation (even if they wanted to), IP theory suggested that attention determined *which* aspects of the situation would enter a person's mind and be retained over time (Atkinson & Schiffrin, 1968). In other words, attention was alleged to be a *precondition* for learning. Quite naturally, teachers familiar with this perspective assumed that their first challenge was to figure out a way to get children to attend to them and not attend to other aspects of the classroom.

One further aspect of attention became evident after IP theorists conducted studies of skill acquisition (Anderson, 1990). Studies showed that when people are first learning a skill, they have to think about what they are doing and frequently talk to themselves. For example, a person learning how to drive a car might say: "Let's see. To put it in reverse, I have to push the stick shift down and to the right . . . I think." But if novices are paying attention to what they are doing, they cannot attend to other aspects of the situation—given the capacity limitations of working memory. It is for this reason that new drivers cannot usually switch gears and participate in a conversation at the same time. Similarly, beginning readers often sound out words properly but fail to comprehend what they are reading. Over time, however, the execution of such skills become increasingly *automatic*, that is, learners can perform these skills without thinking about what they are doing. In this way, working memory capacity is said to be "freed up" by the automatization of skills.

So far, IP theory has been shown to provide explanations of phenomena such as the cocktail party effect, the selectivity of encoding, and the ability of experts to attend to other things besides the execution of skills. But, as I noted in Chapter 3, theories also provide a service by specifying the way in which an ability should be decomposed (or "carved") into elements. One hallmark of the IP approach is the use of so-called rational task analysis (RTA) to determine the components of some ability (e.g., Newell & Simon, 1972). In RTA, a theorist considers the kinds of operations that an ability clearly must involve for logical reasons. To illustrate, RTA suggests that chess ability has to at least involve knowledge of the rules of the game (component 1) and the ability to think several moves ahead (component 2).

In the case of visual attention, RTA suggests the following kinds of component operations (Posner, 1995; Posner & Raichle, 1994). First, a person has to able to maintain a reasonable state of *alertness* and *arousal* in order to detect changes in a situation. Students who fail to get enough sleep often find themselves a few steps behind their fellows. Second, a person has to be able to *disengage* attention from the current stimulus (e.g, stop reading or working intently on something to focus instead on new directions given by a teacher). Third, the person has to be able to *shift* his or her attention to a new stimulus (e.g., look and listen in the direction of the teacher). Fourth, the person has to be able to *discriminate* between the target (e.g., the teacher) and nontargets (e.g., other students in class). Fifth, the person has to be able to *enhance* his or her attention on the focal object. For example, a student has to really listen and concentrate—not just look at the teacher. Sixth, and finally, the person has to be able to *maintain* his or her focus on some target in the face of distractions (e.g., other sounds in the room) and fatigue.

Such an analysis provides useful guidelines as to where to look for individual and developmental differences in attention. For example, perhaps children are similar to adults in their ability to orient, but children may have more trouble than adults when it comes to disengaging attention or maintaining it in the face of distractions. Similarly, perhaps individuals with attention deficits have trouble maintaining attention but do not have trouble orienting toward a new stimulus. Besides providing such guidelines to developmentalists and individual-difference theorists, the RTA of attention can also be useful to neuroscientists who wish to locate brain areas associated with the component operations of attention (as we shall see later; Posner & Raichle, 1994).

The Life-Span View

Life-span theorists examine the development of psychological phenomena from the prenatal period to senescence. The standard approach consists of three elements: (1) decomposing a psychological entity into a set of components, (2) considering whether age changes impact the operation of these components, and (3) proposing developmental mechanisms that can explain any age changes that are observed. In keeping with this general approach, Plude, Enns, and Brodeur (1994) proposed that selective attention is organized around four processes—orienting, filtering, searching, and expecting—and then reviewed the developmental literature to see whether there are age changes in any of these processes.

The first process, *orienting*, involves the alignment of sensory receptors with specific locations in space (Plude et al., 1994). A primitive kind of orienting called the *orienting reflex* is evident in the tendency to automatically shift attention to changes in the environment. When a student comes late to class, for example, most other students demonstrate the orienting reflex by turning their heads toward the person walking in.

Unfortunately for the teacher, most students simultaneously tune out what the teacher is saying until the tardy person sits down. Of course, in addition to such overt kinds of orienting, there are also more covert kinds. For example, airline passengers can usually shift their attention away from a book they are reading to attend to an interesting conversation across the aisle without moving their heads or letting on that they are listening.

Research on the various kinds of orienting shows very little evidence of developmental change from infancy to old age. For example, studies show that even newborns have the orienting reflex. Indeed, by 1 month of age, infants demonstrate the additional tendency to become so captivated by certain stimuli that they cry because they cannot stop looking. Fortunately, infants gain the ability to disengage their attention by the end of the first year. After that point, no substantial age changes are found in orienting, even when the elderly are compared to younger subjects (Plude et al., 1994).

The second process, *filtering*, is the ability to focus on certain attributes of a stimulus to the exclusion of others. As illustrated in dichotic listening tasks and visual discrimination tasks, filtering requires the ability to avoid being distracted by extraneous stimuli (e.g., the content of a conversation while working on a task in the classroom or the library). Developmental studies have revealed a pattern of increasing control over this form of selective attention from childhood to early adulthood. In addition, studies have shown that young children and the elderly are much more likely to fall prey to involuntary perceptual intrusions and behavioral responses than older children, adolescents, and young adults. Whereas the performance of the elderly can be enhanced through various scaffolds, researchers have found it nearly impossible to diminish filtering problems in young children (Plude et al., 1994). As I hinted earlier, perhaps this change reflects brain development.

The third process, *searching*, is exemplified by the situation in which a person leaves a shopping mall and attempts to locate his or her car in the parking lot. In this and similar situations, the person engages in visual scanning of a defined spatial area and then zeros in on certain objects that match the target in global (e.g., shape and color) and specific ways (e.g., license plates). Obviously, this form of selective attention requires an analysis of details and a systematic, thorough approach. Studies have found fairly consistent age changes in searching throughout early childhood. After that point, few age differences are observed, though decrements in scanning have sometimes been found in studies of the elderly (Plude et al., 1994).

The fourth process, *expecting*, goes beyond the ability to shift attention to conspicuous objects (orienting), focus on certain stimuli to the exclusion of others (filtering), and locate important objects (searching). Expectant attention involves the use of environmental cues to be more prepared to process some target object. Two kinds of expectant attention situations have been examined in developmental studies: priming and prompting (Plude et al., 1994). In priming situations, a stimulus (e.g., an arrow on a screen) indicates the likely location of a target (e.g., a letter). In prompting situations, a prior stimulus is either in the same or in a different category as a later stimulus. In making same–different judgments, a person has to rely on information stored in memory. As the amount of time increases between presentation of the cue and the response, memory demands increase as well.

Developmental studies suggest that priming effects can be observed in children as young as 6. However, older children show more efficient use of cues than younger children. Whereas few differences have been observed between the elderly and younger subjects for priming effects, the elderly are similar to young children in their difficulty with memory-demanding tasks (Plude et al, 1994).

The literature as a whole, then, shows that age changes only emerge for certain kinds of attentional processes. In addition, the research generally supports two main conclusions. First, the aspects of attention that change the most during the early part of life are also those that decline the most at the end of life. Second, the attentional tasks that are hardest for young adults (because they require strategies and a certain amount of cognitive effort) are also the ones that show the greatest change between childhood, adulthood, and old age (Plude et al., 1994).

The Vygotskian View

The noted Russian psychologist Lev Vygotsky believed that there were two kinds of attention: natural and higher order (Vygotsky, 1978). *Natural attention* was said to be involuntary and closely linked to immediate perception. *Higher order attention*, in contrast, was said to be voluntary, symbolic, and strategic. Vygotsky proposed that during development, most children shift from relying exclusively on natural attention to relying on both kinds of attention. The key event that facilitates this transition, he argued, is the internalization of language. Internalized language helps children to think of perceptual scenes as integrated wholes, and to think of objects as falling into certain categories. In addition, language helps children and adults extend their thinking back into the past and forward into the future. As such, they can bring their past experiences to bear on the current situation, as well as engage in planning. Further, one form of language called *inner speech* helps children to regulate and control their behaviors (including their attentional focus), and avoid being distracted.

Although Vygotsky acknowledged various forms of communication in nonhuman species, he argued that the internalization of *human* language is a necessary precondition for the development of higher order attention. As such, he assumed that young children (who have not completely internalized language) are similar to animals in their reliance on the natural, involuntary kind of attention. Note that this explanation differs from a more biologically based one (unless one assumes that the internalization process is constrained by brain development).

The Emergent Motivation View

Readers of this book can probably identify situations in which they were so engrossed in an activity that they lost all sense of time and place. Such situations have been dubbed "flow" experiences by motivation researchers (Csikszentmihalyi, 1998). These experiences are said to occur most often during activities that allow for free expression and creativity, such as games, play, and art (Pintrich & Schunk, 1996). Obviously, flow experiences are relevant to the psychology of selective attention because they involve focusing on certain things to the exclusion of others. In addition, it can be argued that the motivational construct of interest is also relevant to attention given the fact that interest often determines what we attend to in particular situations. For some reason, however, the links between motivation and attention have rarely been explored by psychologists who approach attention from the IP, life-span, or Vygotskian perspectives.

The "Flashbulb" Memory Phenomenon

In addition to flow experiences, readers of this book can also probably identify personal experiences that seem to be permanently burned into their memories. For example, most people remember where they were when they heard about the *Challenger* disaster (or the Kennedy assassination, in the case of baby boomers). These experiences stand out in people's minds because of the unusual level of detail that is retained. Why do we remember so much about these experiences and so little about others?

One possibility is that we tend to be fully engaged in such emotionally charged situations (a point discussed further in Chapter 5). In other words, nearly all of our attentional resources are devoted to encoding the event. Another possibility is that we tend to replay the event over and over in our minds and also repeatedly discuss details with friends (thereby making use of rehearsal mechanisms—see Chapter 3). A third possibility is that we create very elaborate encodings of these situations because they evoke so many thoughts (which also enhance memory—see Chapter 3). There are, of course, neuroscientific explanations of the flashbulb phenomenon as well. These will be discussed later in this chapter.

The Educational Perspective

In Chapter 3, we learned that people are more likely to remember information if they actively process this information than if they passively process it (i.e., the so-called generation effect). Some educational researchers (e.g., Wittrock, 1991) have argued that active processing promotes greater retention because it fosters enhanced attention to the to-be-learned material. Examples of active processing include making up sentences when studying vocabulary words, thinking of analogies when studying science concepts, and making up math problems for fellow students. Many cognitive psychologists attribute the generation effect to the fact that it involves elaborative encoding. However, the claim that it also involves attention and the neural substrates of attention is worth consideration.

The Clinical Perspective

In recent years, there has been intense interest in the disorder known as attention-deficit/hyperactivity disorder (ADHD). ADHD is believed to occur in 3–7% of the population, though boys are three times more likely to be diagnosed with this disorder than girls (Barkley, 1997). The fourth edition of the *Diagnostic and Statistical Manual of Mental Disorders* (DSM-IV; American Psychiatric Association, 1994) specifies that there are three subtypes of ADHD: the predominantly inattentive type, the predominantly hyperactive–impulsive type, and the combined type.

Licensed clinicians assign the predominantly inattentive type when a child or adult demonstrates six or more of the following symptoms for at least 6 months to a degree that is maladaptive and inconsistent with developmental level: (1) often fails to give close attention to details or makes careless mistakes in schoolwork, work, or other activities; (2) often has difficulty sustaining attention in tasks or play activities; (3) often does not seem to listen when spoken to directly; (4) often does not follow through or finish schoolwork, chores, or duties in the workplace; (5) often has difficulty organizing activities; (6) often avoids tasks that require sustained mental effort; (7) often loses things that are necessary for tasks; (8) often is easily distracted by extraneous stimuli; and (9) often is forgetful in daily activities.

The predominantly hyperactive–impulsive type is assigned when a child or adult demonstrates six or more of the following symptoms for at least 6 months to a degree that is maladaptive and inconsistent with developmental level: (1) often fidgets or squirms; (2) often leaves seat in situations requiring one to stay seated; (3) often runs about or climbs in situations where such behaviors are inappropriate; (4) often has difficulty engaging in quiet leisure activities; (5) often is "on the go" or seems to be "driven by a motor"; (6) often talks excessively; (7) often blurts out answers before questions have been completed; (8) often has difficulty waiting for his or her turn; and (9) often interrupts or intrudes on others.

The combined type of ADHD is to be assigned when six or more of the criteria for both inattention and hyperactivity–impulsivity have been met. For all three types, however, the DSM-IV suggests that the diagnosis is more likely to be given when some of the symptoms causing impairment have been present before the age of 7 years, the symptoms appear in at least two settings (e.g., school and home), and no other major disorder involving attention or impulse problems is present (e.g., schizophrenia or conduct disorder). Recent studies, however, have questioned use of the age-of-onset criterion because it fails to adequately account for the large proportion of individuals who manifest the disorder (especially attention problems) or after age 7 (Barkley & Bierderman, 1997; Applegate et al., 1997).

In the present context, only the first and third types of ADHD are of interest, given the symptoms associated with attention problems. Although it is generally believed that this disorder has an organic origin (given the fact that certain caffeine-like medications apparently help sometimes), note that the symptomatology of the DSM-IV is entirely behavioral. Hence, it seems appropriate to characterize the clinical perspective as being a psychological perspective rather than a neuroscientific perspective. The neuropsychology of ADHD will, however, be addressed later in this chapter.

Before moving on to the neuroscientific perspectives, it is worth noting that ADHD probably represents the low end of a continuum of attentional and impulse-control problems. Everyone "spaces out," loses things, and acts impulsively sometimes. The issue is whether these symptoms can be controlled by the individual (through strategies, increased effort, etc.), whether they happen more often than not, and whether they cause serious problems in school or at work.

NEUROSCIENTIFIC PERSPECTIVES ON ATTENTION

As was the case for psychologists, neuroscientists have approached the topic of attention from a variety of perspectives. One strand of research arose in response to the suggestion that attention helps animals (including humans) behave adaptively in particular situations (Posner, 1995). Other strands arose in response to analyses of fascinating case studies of brain-injured individuals. In a recent attempt to integrate these various perspectives, Posner (1995) proposed that the anatomy of attention is comprised of three interrelated networks that support distinct cognitive functions. After I describe Posner's account, I shall explore an alternative account as well as other neuroscientific issues related to the constructs of arousal and ADHD.

Posner's Attentional Network Account

Posner and colleagues (e.g., Posner, 1995; Posner & Raichle, 1994) argue that there appear to be three brain-based attentional networks: an orienting network, an executive network, and an alerting network. The primary role of the *orienting network* is to help animals shift attention to changes in the environment. Such a network would obviously involve any brain structures that allow an animal to look or listen in the direction of the change (e.g., centers that control the movement of the head, ears, and eyes), but this network has also been shown to involve structures associated with more covert shifts of attention. As I noted earlier, humans and nonhuman animals respond more rapidly and accurately when given cues as to the likely location of some target. In experiments involving such cues, electrical recordings taken at the scalp and intracellular recordings of single brain cells show evidence of increased efficiency well before the eyes begin to move (Posner, 1995).

Studies of brain-injured individuals and surgically altered animals suggest that the parietal lobes (especially the right one) are associated with the ability to disengage attention from its present focus. Damage to this area results in the problem of being "glued" to a particular stimulus. Perhaps it is the immaturity of the parietal lobes that explains the tendency of 1-month-old infants to be similarly glued to a stimulus (as I noted earlier). If all goes well with the disengagement process, the next step is to move the center of attention to the area of the target. The *supe-*

rior colliculus and surrounding midbrain areas seem to be important structures for this shift of attention (see Figure 1.2). Finally, the *pulvinar nucleus* of the thalamus seems to be important to the process of filtering out irrelevant stimuli (Posner, 1995).

A protracted controversy in the psychology of attention focuses on whether selective attention operates in the early stages of information processing or whether it occurs relatively late, after the majority of potentially relevant stimuli have been analyzed at a fairly high level (Posner, 1995; Hillyard, Mangun, Woldorff, & Luck, 1995). Traditional psychological measures (e.g., reaction time) have not been very useful for resolving this controversy. In recent years, however, researchers have made use of the excellent temporal resolution properties of EEGs and ERPs to provide evidence in favor of the early selection views. Given the equivocal nature of the latter kind of measures (see Chapter 1), however, it should not be surprising to learn that some psychologists do not agree that the early–late controversy has been resolved (Hillyard et al., 1995). An additional problem is that the EEG approach is currently incapable of determining whether stimulus filtering occurs primarily in the thalamus or in cortical areas.

Posner and colleagues suggest that after the orienting network completes its task of locating a change in the environment, the *executive network* becomes operative. RTA suggests that there must be some attentional network that helps people go beyond mere awareness that an object is present. People also have to be able to determine the category of an object (to know if it is the kind of object that they are looking for), and, more generally, to know whether their goal of finding an object has been met (Posner & Raichle, 1994). The executive network, if it exists, must involve all the brain structures that are associated with target detection, including those associated with categorization, working memory, and fulfilling goals or instructions. This network also probably involves structures associated with voluntary control over attention and the ability to inhibit responses to nontargets.

The *anterior cingulate gyrus* (see Figure 1.2) is thought to be the key brain structure in the executive network for several reasons (Posner & Raichle, 1994). First, it has direct anatomical connections to structures involved in semantic memory, working memory, inhibition, and goal-directed behaviors. Second, neuroimaging studies have found that the vast majority of target detection tasks (regardless of content) activate this structure. In fact, most studies show that as the number of targets increases, so does the level of activation of the anterior cingulate. Third, bilateral damage to this structure sometimes results in a condition in which people fail to initiate voluntary activity for some period of time (*akinetic mutism*).

The third attentional network is called the *vigilance network* because it is operative in situations in which a person must remain alert as he or she waits for the occurrence of some event (Posner, 1995; Posner & Raichle, 1994). This network would obviously be useful for military personnel or air traffic controllers who monitor radar screens, but it also would be useful for ordinary individuals doing mundane things such as waiting to hear signs that an infant is waking up from a nap. Neuroimaging studies suggest that regions of the right parietal and right frontal lobes are especially active when a person has to maintain a vigilant state. Interestingly, the anterior cingulate is not active when these two regions are active. In addition, studies show that an individual's heart rate slows when these regions are active.

Aston-Jones et al.'s Attentional Model

Whereas Posner and colleagues assume that the thalamus plays a key role in selective attention and that the vigilance aspect is mediated by parietal and frontal structures, Aston-Jones and colleagues (e.g., Aston-Jones, Rajkowski, & Cohen, 1999) argue that the *locus ceruleus* (LC), a structure somewhat inferior to the thalamus (located in the fourth ventricle of the brainstem), is responsible for both aspects of attention. They base their claim on several facts. First, this nucleus innervates and projects to a greater variety of brain areas than any other single nucleus yet described. Second, there are particularly dense LC projections to areas that are associated with attentional processing (i.e., the parietal cortex, pulvinar nucleus, and superior colliculus). Third, norepinephrine (NE) projections from the LC have been found to augment evoked activity (either excitatory or inhibitory) in neurons while decreasing their spontaneous activity. This action is thought to bring about an enhanced signal-to-noise ratio in target systems. Fourth, tonic activity in the NE projections has been found to vary according to sleepiness and arousal. Finally, single-unit recording of neurons in the LC have shown that these neurons are selectively responsive to target stimuli. For example, monkeys trained to press a lever when a horizontal line appears but not when a vertical line appears show a high level of activity in the LC neurons only when the horizontal line appears.

The Neuroscientific Basis of Arousal Effects

Neuroscientists have been interested in the construct of arousal for over 40 years. To a large extent, this interest grew out of desire to understand the anatomical basis of the effect of stress on memory (Cahill & McGaugh, 1998; Robbins & Everitt, 1995). Beginning with Yerkes and

Dodson (1908), it has been argued that animals seem to learn more when they are in a state of moderate arousal than when they are in states of either low arousal or high arousal (an inverted-U-shaped learning curve). Placed in a classroom context, this finding suggests that students are more likely to learn material if they are moderately stressed (by a moderately demanding or moderately intimidating teacher) than if they are extremely anxious or only slightly anxious. Over the years, neuroscientists have advanced a number of proposals regarding the neuroscientific basis of this phenomenon. Recent proposals have emphasized the roles of hormones released in the periphery as well as distinct tracts of neurons in the brain.

Regarding the first proposal, the adrenal glands (situated on top of the kidneys) release both epinephrine ("adrenaline") and norepinephrine during stressful situations. Among other things, the former acts to dilate the pupils, increase heart rates, and constrict blood vessels. Neither hormone, however, crosses the blood–brain barrier, so it was generally assumed that neither could play a significant role in the stress modulation of memory. However, recent studies show that the standard effects of stress on memory can be eliminated by administering substances that block the action of these two adrenomedullary hormones (Cahill & McGaugh, 1998). Thus, epinephrine and norepinephrine must play some sort of role. One proposal that has gained empirical support in recent years is the idea that epinephrine affects memory through its modulation of glucose levels in the blood. Glucose levels have also been found to be linked to learning in an inverted-U-shaped manner (i.e., medium levels promote more learning than low or high levels), and the level of epinephrine in the blood affects the level of glucose in the blood (Cahill & McGaugh, 1998). An alternative is to assume that another adrenal hormone, cortisol, not epinephrine or norepinephrine, is responsible for stress-related effects on memory. The hippocampus has receptors for cortisol, a substance that has been found to cause memory problems when it is acutely administered (Sapolsky, 1999; Schmidt, Fox, Goldberg, Smith, & Schulkin, 1999).

Regarding the second proposal, dopaminergic (DA) neurons that connect the amygdala to the frontal lobes have been found to be activated under stressful situations (Cahill & McGaugh, 1998). As will be discussed in Chapter 5, the amygdala is thought to be an important structure for negative emotions such as fear and anger. In Chapter 3, we learned that the frontal lobes are important for working memory, so the idea that dopaminergic neurons might be involved appears to have some merit.

Other neural tracts that seem to affect arousal include the noradrenergic (NA) tract of the LC that extends to distinct forebrain regions, the DA tract that extends from the midbrain to the ventral striatum and anterior neocortex, the cholinergic tract that extends from the brainstem to structures such as the prefrontal cortex and the thalamus, and the serotonin (5-HT) tract that extends from the raphe nuclei of the midbrain to many of the same regions innervated by the NA tract (Robbins & Everitt, 1995). A combination of pharmacological, surgical, and clinical case studies suggests that the NA system helps animals to maintain stimulus discriminations in the midst of stressful situations. The DA system, in contrast, seems to play a role in the activation of motoric and cognitive outputs. The cholinergic system seems to function to enhance processing at the cortical level, and the 5-HT system apparently dampens the effects of the other systems through its inhibitory and dearousing effects.

The Neuroscientific Basis of ADHD

One strand of neuroscientific research that is also worth considering is that pertaining to ADHD. The first step in identifying the brain structures associated with ADHD is to have a clear and consistent definition of this disorder. In other words, it makes little sense to compare brain structures and functions in ADHD and non-ADHD groups when it is not clear that the people in each group really belong in that group. Although the empirically derived DSM-IV definition goes a long way in clarifying the issue, there are certain points of vagueness in this definition that could cause diagnostic problems. For example, at what age is inattention or impulsivity developmentally inappropriate (Barkley, 1997)? Is it when a child is 5 or when he or she is 7 or 8? Similarly, at what point are attentional problems so severe that they are maladaptive? Is it when an intelligent child earns "C" grades in school or when this child regularly gets sent to the principal? These points of vagueness imply that any neuroscientific study of ADHD is open to multiple interpretations.

Moreover, even if we were to suspend concerns about proper diagnosis, there is still the problem that technologies such as fMRI have only become widely available in recent years. It is for these reasons that it is difficult to draw firm conclusions from the extant neuroscientific studies of ADHD. Scientists interested in this issue can turn to the various structures mentioned above in the discussions of Posner's account and the arousal studies. Until these leads are followed, we can only tentatively consider the recent proposal of Barkley (1997) that the predominantly hyperactive–impulsive and combined types of ADHD reflect frontal lobe abnormalities. The frontal lobes are involved in behavioral inhibition and working memory, and children who have been diagnosed with either the hyperactive–impulsive or combined types of ADHD have problems in inhibition and memory. However, it is also possible that subcortical structures are also affected in ADHD, especially in the case of the predominantly inattentive type.

One way to potentially clarify the neuroscientific basis of ADHD is to consider the sites of action of drugs such as Ritalin (methylphenidate). These drugs are clearly overused and only partially effective, but it is nevertheless interesting to note that stimulant drugs seem to target two of the neural tracts described earlier, namely, the DA and NA tracts (Solanto, 1998). The effect of stimulants on the DA tract appears to be improvements in locomotor activity and responsiveness to reinforcement (in the case of rats). The effect of stimulants on the NA tract appears to be improvements in delayed responding and working memory.

CONCLUSIONS, CAVEATS, AND INSTRUCTIONAL IMPLICATIONS

It seems that scientists have learned at least three important things about attention since the time of William James. First, they have learned that the component operations of attention include such things as orienting, filtering, and enhancing. Second, they have learned that attention can be both automatic and controlled. Third, they have learned that some, but not all, of the components of attention change with age. Beyond these general points, however, the present chapter shows that there may be important links between attention, motivation, and emotion, and that there is a fair amount of overlap between the psychological and neuroscientific perspectives on attention.

In retrospect, the overlap between the psychological and neuroscientific perspectives is to be somewhat expected, given the fact that neuroscientists have often used psychological descriptions as "road maps" to find the sites of particular attentional operations (e.g., orienting). Similarly, psychologists have often returned the favor by relying on neuroscientific methods in attempts to resolve several important controversies in the field of attention.

Despite some very clear advances in the field, however, one could argue that there is still much to learn. Some would question, for example, whether scientists have really resolved important controversies through the use of neuroscientific methods (Hillyard et al., 1995). Another problem is that contemporary descriptions of attention are still too vague to be useful to those with applied interests. From an instructional standpoint, for example, we still do not know enough about attention to provide comprehensive answers to basic questions such as the following: (1) How can teachers create learning environments that maximize student attention? and (2) How, exactly, is attention related to learning and retention? Nevertheless, the literature has advanced enough to suggest that teachers can manage attention through the use of content that is interesting to students and by holding moderately high standards for performance (in which students are held accountable for not meeting these standards). Moreover, teachers should establish routines to allow efficient progress toward goals, but then periodically change routines to engage the orienting aspects of attention. Further, students should be asked to be active participants in the learning process and to construct their own understandings.

Notwithstanding these suggestions, one may still wonder why we have not learned more about attention over the past 100 years and why more links to classroom practice have not emerged. One possible explanation is that scientists have spent more time trying to reveal the components of attention than they have trying to understand the causal effects of attention. As a result, they are unable to provide answers to questions such as the following: What happens in our brains when we concentrate and why does concentration seem to lead to better retention? In addition, as I argued in Chapter 1, neuroscientific evidence is primarily useful to the extent that it helps us decide which of two competing theories seems to be more accurate. Accurate theories, in turn, provide the basis for effective instructional practices. In other words, once we know how something (such as attention) works, we can usually figure out how to make it work to our advantage. It can be argued that the neuroscience of attention has not advanced to the point that it can help us decide among competing psychological theories of attention.

And yet the available research on attention is somewhat useful when it is viewed through a developmental lens. As I noted earlier, studies have shown that there are aspects of attention that are particularly hard for children in elementary school (i.e., filtering) and others that are not that hard (i.e., orienting). Clearly, teachers need to take this "natural" distractability into account when they design instructional contexts. A busy, noisy environment is bound to cause problems for children in the early grades. In addition, there is a need to repeatedly remind children of the goals of an activity as well as the instructions for completing an activity. Moreover, knowing that children cannot help being distracted should also reduce the amount of irritation that teachers, parents, and coaches experience. But it is important to note that these implications derive from a psychological account of attention (i.e., the lifespan view), not a neuroscientific account. In the future, it may be shown that developmental trends in attention have a neurological basis (e.g., maturation of the frontal lobes or a frontal–parietal network).

The idea of developmentally appropriate expectations is also relevant to the diagnosis of ADHD. Recall that the definition of ADHD suggests that this disorder is to be assigned when the symptoms are demonstrated to the degree that it is maladaptive and inconsistent with developmental level. Since the average kindergartner, first grader, or second grader is highly distractable, it makes little sense to assign the label of ADHD to any children in these grades. Similarly, when children in these grades are said to be having problems with attention, one can ask whether the child is the problem or the instructional demands of the classroom is the problem. Are they being asked to do too much at once? Is the classroom somewhat chaotic? The diagnosis of ADHD would, however, be appropriate for middle school students who exhibit the attentional skills of younger children. At some point, moreover, it does make sense to require children to stay on task and refrain from engaging in behaviors that are inappropriate for the context (e.g., talking and walking about when they are supposed to be working silently on a classroom task).

In closing, I must note that it would be useful for psychologists and neuroscientists to move beyond the current understanding of attention to address more of the questions raised by practitioners. In addition, research should be conducted to resolve many of the controversies regarding the true nature and causal effects of attention. Finally, it would be important for researchers to reveal the neuroscientific basis of disorders such as ADHD and also resolve discrepancies regarding the regions of the brain that are responsible for attention (Is vigilance mediated by the LC, the parietal lobes, or the frontal lobes?). If scientists could figure out how the brains of individuals with ADHD differ from those without ADHD, it might then become possible to develop more effective ways to treat this disorder. In addition, we would simultaneously gain important new insights into the normal developmental course of attention as well.

CHAPTER 5

Emotion

In Chapter 1, I noted that psychologists and educators fall into two main camps: those who believe that neuroscientific research is relevant to the fields of psychology and education, and those who believe that neuroscientific research is largely irrelevant. In other words, when asked "Do you believe that your understanding of some psychological phenomenon [e.g., learning] would change if you were to read the neuroscientific literature on this phenomenon?," those in the latter camp would probably respond "No." However, I suspect that if these same individuals were to be pressed about the specific case of emotions, many would start to equivocate or shift their response to "Well . . . maybe." Hence, it seems reasonable to suggest that many people are comfortable with the idea that emotions have a physiological basis.

Why are emotions so readily assumed to have a neural basis? One reason might be that emotional experiences tend to involve the whole body. When people are intensely angry, for example, they (1) take on a distinct posture (e.g., tensed arms and legs), (2) make an easy-to-identify anger expression, (3) have a certain tone in their voices, (4) engage in characteristic sorts of behaviors (e.g., door slamming and arm flailing), and (5) have numerous angry thoughts (e.g., "This is the last straw!").

A second reason why emotions seem so neurological is that most people have had so-called flashbulb experiences in which they remember exactly where they were when something upsetting happened (see Chapter 3). In folk psychology terms, emotions seem to "burn" such experiences into their minds.

My primary goal in this chapter is to describe both the psychological and the neuroscientific perspectives on emotion in such a way that the compatibility of these two perspectives can be adequately assessed. My secondary goal is to consider the instructional implications of research on emotions. As in other chapters, I will present the psychological perspective before the neuroscientific perspective.

Before proceeding, however, it is useful to make several introductory comments regarding the role of emotions in classroom learning and behaviors. As many scholars have noted (e.g., Anderson, 1990; Weiner, 1985), human behavior is aptly characterized as being goal-directed. That is, when people behave in a particular context (e.g., fool around in a classroom), they are usually trying to achieve some goal (e.g., win approval from their friends). As we shall see in the next section, our emotions "pull" us toward certain outcomes and "push" us away from others. If this is so, then it is imperative that teachers design classroom environments that (1) align positive emotions (e.g., pride) with achievement behaviors and outcomes (e.g., mastery over some content) and (2) align negative emotions (e.g., fear) with behaviors and outcomes that are incompatible with achievement. When emotions and outcomes are not properly aligned (e.g., anxiety is linked to the learning of certain information; children gain substantially more pleasure from impressing friends than from doing well on an assignment), children do not learn nearly as much as they could. Second, emotions are very salient and capture our attention in the same way that a pager or physical aches and pains might. Given that attention is the gateway to learning (see Chapter 4), a misalignment of emotions and classroom tasks would lead to poor learning. Moreover, when emotions are too extreme, they capture too much of children's limited attentional resources and restrict how much they learn in yet another way. In other words, children think about how they are feeling instead of thinking about the content of a classroom exercise. Finally, the phenomenon of flashbulb experiences suggests that emotional reactions may somehow interface with the neurophysiology of learning. For example, substances released during emotional reactions (e.g., neurotransmitters in the brain and stress hormones in the periphery) could speed up, or enhance, the process of synaptogenesis. If this is case (and we still do not know for sure if it is the case), emotions would impact learning by directing students' attention, determining the goals they pursue during a lesson, and enhancing the formation of synapses in some way. Hence, emotions are clearly related to classroom learning.

PSYCHOLOGICAL PERSPECTIVES ON EMOTION

It has taken nearly 100 years for psychologists to reach an apparent consensus regarding the nature and function of emotions in the human mind (see Ekman & Davidson, 1994). To a large extent, however, this consensus is more implicit than explicit, given the fact that scholars in this area still disagree about several important issues (LeDoux, 1995). Nevertheless, comparison of prominent models of emotion reveals that these models are based on a number of common assumptions. In what follows, I describe three of these models to illustrate this convergence of perspectives. Then I consider several important issues in the development of emotions.

Three Contemporary Models of Emotion

Although a number of theories of emotion have been proposed over the years, one could argue that the following models are currently the most influential:

Frijda's Model

According in Nico Frijda, emotions involve an appraisal component and a response component (Frijda, 1994). The *appraisal component* operates as a signaling device to inform a person's cognitive and action systems that something has occurred that has relevance to the person's concerns or well-being. In other words, if an event elicits an emotion in people, there must be something in the situation that leads them to expect that they will be either helped or hindered in their pursuit of their goals. To illustrate this basic idea, note that people are naturally concerned about being hurt or killed. Frijda suggests that fear is our mind's way of telling us that something harmful is present in the current situation (or will be present soon). Some of the environmental cues that could elicit fear include such things as (1) objects moving quickly toward us, (2) very steep drops below us, and (3) unexpected loud noises.

Frijda (1994) elaborated on this core proposal by noting that positive emotions tend to be elicited by events that do one of three things: satisfy some motive or goal (e.g., hope, joy), enhance a person's chances of survival (e.g., attachment, love), or demonstrate a person's abilities (e.g., pride, satisfaction). Negative emotions, in contrast, signal to the action system that something should be done to correct a problem (e.g., frustration, guilt) or prevent undesirable things from happening (e.g., fear, anger). In essence, the claim is that "the ends are what give the emotional event its emotional valence" (p. 113). Metaphorically, the positive emotions can be thought of as "pushing" people toward the ends they desire and "pulling" them away from the ends they do not desire (Frijda, 1994). It is clearly adaptive to have a built-in alerting system that tells people that there are conditions present that could either facilitate or impede the attainment of their goals (including their survival).

But being alerted to relevant events is only part of the story. Adaptation requires that an organism initiate a set of actions that could provide an appropriate response to the signal (the *response component* of emotions). For example, an adaptive response to the experience of fear (appraisal component) might be to run away (response component). Similarly, an adaptive response to feeling frustrated when confronted with an obstacle (e.g., a traffic jam), is to do an "end run" around the obstacle or to double one's efforts. Hence, emotions serve to motivate a set of behaviors that could deal effectively with a goal-related event.

In saying that emotions operate as a kind of relevance-signaling system, Frijda (1994) suggests that emotions play a communicative role *within a person*. But he adds that emotions can also play a communicative role *within a group*. Note that all the basic emotions (i.e., fear, anger, joy, sadness, etc.) involve a characteristic facial expression that people can readily identify (Ekman, 1994). These expressions combined with appropriate responses (e.g., shrieking and running in the case of fear) tell others that something of concern has appeared in the immediate environment. Thus, even if only one animal in a group has seen or smelled something ominous, the others nearby can be appropriately alerted by the behavior of the individual who has sensed something. In an analogous way, all the other emotions can be shown to foster appropriate social responses. Note, for example, how people in a group react when someone in their midst has a facial expression indicating sadness, anger, or embarrassment. At a general level, emotions are thought to regulate a group and to promote the group's survival.

Clore's Model

Gerald Clore (1994) suggests that there are three broad classes of emotions that can be distinguished in terms of their focus. Whereas emotions in the first class focus on the *outcomes of events*, emotions in the second and third classes focus on the *agency of actions* and the *attributes of objects*, respectively. If people focus on the outcomes of events (Class 1), they will either be *pleased* or *displeased* with these outcomes (depending on their goals). For example, people feel joy when their favorite team wins a championship, but feel disappointed and dejected when their team loses. To be able to feel pleased or displeased, a person has to appraise outcomes as being either *desirable* or *undesirable*. The emotions in Class 1 include hope, fear, relief, disappointment, happiness, and sadness.

If people focus on the agency of actions (Class 2), they can either *approve* or *disapprove* of these actions. A minimal requirement for being able to approve or disapprove of an action is to have some sort of internal *standard* against which the action could be judged (Clore, 1994). Emotions are elicited in this category when actions are appraised as being either *praiseworthy* or *blameworthy*, relative to the internal standard. For example, a sports fan might feel pride if his or her team played at a particularly high level. Emotions such as guilt or embarrassment reflect similar kinds of standards-based reasoning. The emotions in Class 2 include pride, shame, guilt, embarrassment, admiration, and reproach.

If people focus on the attributes of objects (Class 3), they will either find these attributes *appealing* or *unappealing*. The relative appealingness of attributes is a reflection of an individual's attitudes (Clore, 1994). Examples of emotions in this category include love, hate, and disgust. According to this view, people do not feel love because some goal has been attained (Class 1) or because of the praiseworthiness of the loved one's accomplishments (Class 2). Rather, love is felt because the loved one is appealing in a variety of other ways. Disgust is likewise more related to the inherent unappealing qualities of some object (what it looks like or smells like) than to goal pursuit (Class 1) or deviations from some standard (Class 2). In this vein, it is interesting to note that the vast majority of authentic disgust reactions arise from the products of living or decaying animals such as feces or pus (Pinker, 1997). Disgust, then, can be said to be an adaptive avoidance response that protects the individual from the illnesses that could arise from coming in contact with such products.

Clore further assumes that there can be complex emotions that reflect combinations of the three kinds of foci. To illustrate, consider the case of anger. People feel angry when (1) they are displeased about the consequences of events, particularly as these relate to their personal well-being (a Class 1 focus), and (2) they attribute a causal role to the actions of some individual who is thought to be responsible for the injurious outcome (a Class 2 focus). Other examples of multifocus emotions include gratification, gratitude, and remorse.

In line with Frijda (1994), Clore (1994) believes that the primary function of emotion is to provide information: "Emotions supply information to others through distinctive facial and vocal expressions and to oneself through distinctive thoughts and feelings. . . . [They serve] as data for judgment and decision-making . . . and also for reordering processing priorities" (pp. 103–105). The concept of reordered priorities means that people attend to the important things in a situation before they attend to other less important things. Emotions are linked to goals

and values (or *concerns*, as Frijda put it), so they helps us give prece-
dence to emergencies when they arise (as when a father stops mowing a
lawn when he sees his 2-year-old walk out into the street).

One final set of predictions from the model relates to the construct
of emotional intensity. Scientists and nonscientists alike agree that emotions can be experienced in more or in less intense ways. For example,
sometimes we feel a little angry, but other times we feel very angry. To
explain such variations, Clore (1994) suggests that *local variables*, such
as the perceived likelihood of an outcome or the expected degree of devi-
ation from the norm, govern the strength of our emotional reactions. For
example, if a harmful event is extremely likely to occur, we tend to feel
more frightened than if it is not very likely to occur. With respect to actions, we often vary our assessment of praiseworthiness according to
what we expect an individual to be capable of. For example, little children are held less responsible for their actions than older children, so
they tend to evoke less anger in their parents when they transgress (Dix,
Ruble, Grusec, & Nixon, 1986). Relatedly, sports writers and fans tend
to be more amazed when an older athlete returns to top form than when
a struggling younger player does so.

Lazarus's Model

The fundamental construct in Richard Lazarus's model is the idea that
emotions derive from an individual's appraisal of his or her relationship
with the environment (Lazarus, 1991). More specifically, each emotion
is distinguished by it own pattern of primary and secondary appraisal
components. *Primary appraisal* components include goal relevance, goal
congruency, and type of ego involvement. *Secondary appraisal* components include blame or credit, coping potential, and future expectations.
Together, components in these two categories determine an emotion's
core relational theme (CRT), which represents an individual's understanding of the harms and benefits inherent in a particular person–
environment relationship.

This general approach can be illustrated using several goal-
incongruent (negative) and several goal-congruent (positive) emotions.
Lazarus (1991) argues that anger and fright-anxiety are two goal-
incongruent emotions that have distinctive CRTs and action tendencies.
In the case of anger, the CRT is a *demeaning offense against me and
mine*. If during the appraisal of a situation a person feels that he or she
has been the victim of an act that could be called a slight, inconsiderate,
arbitrary, or malevolent, he or she usually becomes angry.

This anger-inducing appraisal results from the following primary and secondary components. First, there must be some goal at stake (e.g., a desire to get a promotion at work). However, having a goal merely sets the condition for any positive or negative emotion, including anger, to be elicited. Second, the event has to be judged to be goal-incongruent (e.g., a boss passes up an employee and promotes a colleague instead). When an event is appraised as being goal-incongruent, only the negative emotions (including anger) are possible. Third, there has to be a threat to one's self-esteem or sense of worth (e.g., being offended at being passed up). This third kind of appraisal narrows the field down further to emotions such as anger, anxiety, and pride.

In order to distinguish among the latter three, it is necessary to invoke the secondary appraisal components. In the case of anger, someone has to be judged responsible for the offense. Note how an unintended and unavoidable offense would not necessarily lead to anger. Next, there must be an appraisal that the demeaning offense is best remedied by an attack. Finally, there needs to be an expectation that the attack would not bring retaliation, punishment, or irreparable damage to a relationship. Thus, anger leads to the potentiation of retaliatory actions. Students prone to violence in the classroom tend to have distorted appraisal processes (e.g., they think that an accidental bump in a crowded hallway was intentional) as well as little inhibitory control over the desire to retaliate (Garber & Dodge, 1991).

Turning next to the example of fright-anxiety, the CRT for fright is *imminent physical harm*; the CRT for anxiety is *uncertain, existential threat*. Both are evoked by events that are relevant to, but incompatible with, a person's goals (similar to anger). If the threat is concrete and centered on bodily harm, fright is experienced. However, if the threat is to one's ego integrity (or self-esteem) and the source is unknown, anxiety develops. Lazarus (1991) argues that the three kinds of secondary appraisal (i.e., blame, coping potential, and future expectation) are largely irrelevant to feelings of fright or anxiety. As for action tendencies, both fright and anxiety are linked to avoidance or escape behaviors. For obvious reasons, teachers would not want their students to develop fear or anxiety reactions to classroom content (e.g., math formulae). They would tend to avoid the content instead of emersing themselves in it to master it.

For two examples of goal-congruent (positive) emotions, we can consider happiness and pride. To experience either of these emotions, events must occur that are judged to be both relevant to and compatible with a person's goals (primary appraisal components 1 and 2). The CRT for happiness is *reasonable progress toward the realization of one's goals*; for pride, it is *enhancement of one's ego identity by taking credit for a valued object or achievement, either our own or that of someone or a group with whom we identify.* As for other appraisal components, Lazarus (1991) argues that type of ego involvement (component 3), blame or credit (component 4), and coping potential (component 5) are all irrelevant to feelings of happiness. Positive future expectations are, however, relevant (component 6). With respect to pride, type of ego involvement and credit (to oneself) are both relevant, but coping potential and future expectations are irrelevant. Lazarus speculates that the action tendency for happiness is expansiveness and outgoingness; for pride, it may be similar kinds of behaviors that often border on bragging or showing off.

Summary

Considered together, all three of the aforementioned psychological theories of emotions assume that emotions have a cognitive aspect that involves considering the relevance of events to one's goals. In addition, emotions are assumed to play a communicative role within and among people. Positive and negative emotions are distinguished in terms of whether the events are judged to be compatible or incompatible with a person's goals. Frijda and Lazarus further assume that emotions are closely linked to specific action tendencies such as attack or escape. Clore, however, suggests that emotions are linked to behaviors by way of decision-making processes and shifts in attention.

The Development of Emotion

As Vygotsky (1978) and many other scholars have noted, the best way to understand the current state of some phenomenon (e.g., emotional expression) is to consider how it emerged from prior states and why it developed in the manner it did. The three models presented in the prior section describe a fully mature system of emotions. Some of the questions that arise in a developmental analysis of emotions include the following:

1. When do children first express and experience various emotions?
2. If some emotions emerge before others, why is this the case?
3. How do the links between the components of emotion (e.g., appraisal and action) change with development?

Charles Darwin was one of the first people to ask and answer such questions. He used his own children as observational subjects. Some 100 years later, researchers rediscovered Darwin's evolutionary approach and developed a sophisticated facial coding system based on it (Izard, 1994). In a recent study that employed this coding system, Izard et al. (1995) found that full-face expressions of interest, joy, sadness, and anger were all present by 2.5 months of age and accounted for 98% of the emotions expressed during the first 9 months of life. However, these results do not necessarily mean that infants in this age range experienced these four emotions in response to appropriate cues in the environment. Camras (1994) reports that infants regularly express facial configurations of surprise and enjoyment in situations that do not call for these emotions, and sometimes fail to express appropriate emotions in situations that do call for them (e.g., a fear expression when approached by a stranger). Thus, one thing that seems to develop in the emotional system is a higher rate of concordance between emotional expressions and cues in the environment. These findings also suggest that the expression component of emotions is in place before the cognitive appraisal component comes on line.

The second important developmental change concerns the conditions or events that elicit emotions (Dunn, 1994). Obviously, what makes an infant or preschooler laugh is not the same as what makes an adolescent or adult laugh. Similarly, young children are afraid of many things that do not frighten older children and adults (e.g., the darkness of their bedrooms). As children's thinking develops and their experiences widen, their appraisals of situations that could invoke laughter or fear (e.g., "that is funny" or "that is scary") change as well. Given the models of emotions presented earlier, another important (but understudied) change would be alterations in children's goals and values (Lazarus, 1994). For example, if young children care more about adults than about their peers, they would not necessarily be afraid to perform, say, a tap dance on stage in front of their peers. By adolescence, however, these same children would probably feel both fear and embarrassment if they were made to perform such a dance in front of their peers.

The third important change concerns children's concept of self and self-esteem. In order for children to experience emotions such as pride, shame, guilt, jealousy, and embarrassment, they need to have a concept of themselves as separate from others as well as to have internalized standards of performance (Dunn, 1994). Most scholars believe that children below the age of 2 do not experience self- and standards-based emotions because they lack a clearly differentiated sense of self and have not yet internalized standards or rules. Taking this analysis one step further, it can be argued that as the sense of self changes between early childhood and late adolescence, emotional responses and eliciting conditions must change as well.

The fourth major developmental trend concerns emotional expressiveness. The human species is said to differ from other animal species in the sense that we sometimes need to hide our emotions in order to adapt to some environmental niche. Adults who "wear their hearts on their sleeve" often fare poorly in the workplace (at least in terms of interpersonal relationships and promotions to leadership positions). As such, children are regularly socialized into "appropriate" forms of expression by their parents and teachers (e.g., big boys don't cry; use your words instead of your fists; etc.) and acquire a large number of natural language labels for emotions that further shape their understanding (Dunn, 1994). The appropriateness of certain expressions would, of course, vary across cultures, as would the number of terms used to denote emotions. As such, one would expect cross-cultural differences in this regard.

The final major developmental change to be discussed has been the subject of a great deal of research in recent years. Children need to learn how to *regulate* their emotions such that they can function adaptively in a variety of situations (Dunn, 1994; Rothbart, 1994). In other words, they need to be able to express positive and negative emotions when these emotions are called for (e.g., at weddings and funerals), and also to inhibit their tendencies to express emotions when restraint is called for (e.g., anger at a boss). In other words, they have to insert a *mediational process* between their appraisals and action tendencies that metaphorically "breaks" the inborn, reflexive link between these two components of emotion. Failure to break the link between certain appraisals (I am being harmed) and certain actions tendencies (I must attack or retaliate) leads to a number of social problems. As I noted earlier, appraisal errors and emotional dysregulation are the key symptoms associated with problems such as social rejection and conduct disorder (Garber & Dodge, 1991; Thompson, 1991).

NEUROSCIENTIFIC PERSPECTIVES ON EMOTION

If neuroscientists were to use the foregoing psychological accounts of emotion as metaphorical "road maps" to help them find functional brain areas associated with emotions, they might try to find one or more brain regions associated with the appraisal process, one or more regions associated with the conscious experience of particular emotions, one or more regions associated with certain action tendencies, as well as possible anatomical evidence for the distinctions among various emotions (e.g., positive vs. negative emotions; pride vs. anger; etc.). For example, several of the models of emotions would gain support if closely related emotions (according to theory) produced similar yet distinct activation patterns in an fMRI study.

It turns out that no one neuroscientist has looked at all the components of emotion in a comprehensive set of studies. Instead, the more common approach is to (1) focus on a few select emotions such as fear or anger, and (2) to study specific issues relevant to these emotions (e.g., identifying the neural pathways of fear). The main reason for this selectivity is that neuroscientists began their work on emotions well before Frijda, Clore, Lazarus, and other researchers proposed comprehensive psychological models. Hence, there were no comprehensive models that could serve as guides (LeDoux, 1995). Another reason is that neuroscientists began their work well before neuroimaging techniques such as PET and fMRI became widely available. As a result, they were often restricted to studying the neural basis of emotions in species such as rats and cats. Use of such species, in turn, restricted the types of emotions that could be studied. Note that rats experience fear but they do not experience pride, guilt, or embarrassment (as far as we know!). In the past few years, however, there has been more of a convergence between the neuroscientific and psychological perspectives as more has become known and neuroimaging techniques have become more accessible.

In what follows, neuroscientific perspectives and research on emotion will be examined in three parts. In the first part, I will focus on several recently proposed neuroscientific models that attempt to summarize several independent stands of research. In the second part, my focus narrows somewhat to specific emotions such as fear and stress-related reactions. In the third part, my focus is on the neuroscientific basis of several emotional deficits.

Three Integrative Perspectives

While it is true that a truly comprehensive and detailed neuroscientific model of emotions has yet to be proposed, several accounts have recently appeared in the literature that extend beyond typical accounts in their scope.

A Network Model of Human Emotions

Halgren and Marinkovic (1995) recently argued that it is possible to integrate three disparate strands of neuroscientific research within a single "network" model. The starting assumption of their model is that there are four successive but overlapping stages in the emotional reaction to some stimulus: (1) the orienting complex, (2), emotional event integration, (3) response selection, and (4) sustained emotional context. The *orienting complex* is an automatic and preconscious response during which a person directs his or her attention toward some event and mobilizes resources for coping with this event. One output of this complex is a neurally encoded stimulus that is passed on to other stages for higher processing. During the second stage, *emotional event integration*, the neurally encoded stimulus is integrated with semantic associates and other information in long-term semantic memory (What kind of event is this and what is its label?), declarative memory (What facts do I know about this event?), and working memory (e.g., aspects of the current context). When the integration is complete, an individual becomes aware of the stimulus, imbues it with a cognitive interpretation and affective tone, and links the event to possible voluntary acts. After a certain amount of deliberation, one of these actions is then chosen during the third stage, *response selection*. In the final stage, *sustained emotional context*, the outputs of the prior stages are linked to, and influenced by, the current "neurophysiological background to phasic events—the subject's mood" (p. 1138).

Halgren and Marinkovic (1995) proposed that each of the four stages is associated with a distinct neural substrate. They based this claim on findings from recording, lesion, and stimulation studies in humans and animals. With respect to the orienting complex, for example, studies with animals and anencephalic infants suggest that the startle and other aspects of the complex are integrated in the midbrain (and possibly the hypothalamus as well). In neurologically intact older humans, this integration results in autonomic activity in the brainstem as well as event-related potentials (ERPs) that can be recorded over the front center of the scalp at 200, 280, and 350 milliseconds after stimulus onset. Further analysis of these ERPs suggested that they appear to be generated by the same parietal–cingulate–dorsolateral circuit that has been identified in studies of directed attention (see Chapter 4).

Psychologists have noted that emotions do more than simply orient attention, so other neural systems must be involved as well. In humans, adaptive responding requires higher level analysis such that distinct subjective experiences and action tendencies are elicited for different emotions and events. Sometimes angry feelings and actions are appropriate, whereas other times happy feelings and actions are appropriate. To know which emotion to evoke, the mind has to engage in emotional event integration (Stage 2). Studies in which the brains of people have been electrically stimulated have found that fear is the most common emotion elicited by direct stimulation of the amygdala (Halgren & Marinkovic, 1995). Amygdalal and hippocampal stimulation has also been found to evoke cardiac and respiratory phenomena. Stimulation of the anterior cingulate gyrus (which also has been found to be active in executive attention; see Chapter 4) elicits equal numbers of positive and negative emotions. Pleasurable feelings can also be evoked by stimulating callosal fibers that are thought to interconnect the posterior orbital and anterior gingulate cortices. Stimulation of the medial temporal lobe has been found to evoke the epigastric sensation that usually rises up from the stomach to the chest and on to the throat and head.

The results of electrical recording studies are generally consistent with those of direct stimulation studies. In particular, there is an ERP called N4/P3b that is generated in multiple association cortex areas (e.g., the fusiform gyrus and superior temporal sulcus) and limbic areas (e.g., the amygdala, hippocampus, and lateral orbitofrontal cortex). The former areas are thought to supply information regarding emotional facial expressions and semantic associates. The latter are thought to provide an emotional evaluation of the presented stimulus and a psychosocial context for encoding it (Halgren & Marinkovic, 1995). The N4 component is a negative component that occurs at about 400 milliseconds and is generated by any potentially meaningful stimulus. Hence, it can be recorded near any site of knowledge storage in the cortex (see Chapter 3). The P3b is a positive component that occurs after excitation has spread information broadly and is thought to reflect the onset of inhibitory processes to dampen inappropriate associations.

As for response selection (Stage 3), the key structures appear to be the supplementary motor cortex and central cingulate gyrus, because (1) lesions in these areas can affect voluntary movement and (2) these areas are metabolically very active when subjects are asked to plan voluntary movements. Finally, sustained emotional context (Stage 4) has been associated with sustained specific firing in distinct areas of the frontal lobe (Halgren & Marinkovic, 1995).

Polyvagal Theory

Porges (1995) recently proposed a model of emotional and attentive functioning that is based on insights gained from Darwinian theory and psychophysiological studies of neural functioning in various phylogenic species. The theory proposes that through evolution, mammals developed two neural subsystems of the vagus nerve (which extend from the brain down to peripheral structures like the heart) to regulate the heart and instigate other adaptive behaviors such as the orienting reflex, increased attention, facial expressions, vocalization, and fight-or-flight responses. Reptiles, in contrast, rely on a single system that exists to support their tendency to simply orient and freeze. Because reptiles have relatively low metabolic demands, their more primitive system instigates an increase in cardiac functioning when they are confronted with a novel or frightening stimulus. Because the metabolic demands of mammals are four to five times higher than those of reptiles, a similar increase in vagal tone during stress would be lethal. As a result, mammals demonstrate a characteristic reduction in vagal tone when exhibiting the orienting reflex that is followed sometime later by a return to baseline.

To explain the link between the vagal system and emotion, Porges (1995) followed Darwin and many others in making a distinction between primary (basic) emotions and culturally based emotions. The primary emotions, which include anger, fear, panic, sadness, surprise, interest, happiness, and disgust, are thought to have an innate neural basis and characteristic corresponding facial expression. Next, he suggested that it is not coincidental that the vagus and basic emotions have an alleged right hemisphere bias. The functional dominance of the right side of the brain in regulating autonomic function and primary emotions allows the left side to gain dominance of motor and language skills (in right-handed individuals). This hemispheric distribution would allow simultaneous activation of functions associated with emotional–homeostatic processes and language–voluntary processes. By implication, this account suggests that shifts in affective states would parallel changes in vagal tone. For example, it would be expected that when a negative emotion is elicited, there would be a withdrawal of vagal tone to promote fight-or-flight behaviors. In a provocative follow-up analysis, Porges (1998) extended this polyvagal account to show how love is an emergent property of the mammalian autonomic nervous system.

Hemispheric Asymmetry Models

Whereas Porges (1995) suggested that all primary emotions are regulated by the right hemisphere, Davidson (1992) and Fox (1991) have advanced proposals suggesting that there is an asymmetric distribution of positive and negative emotions in both hemispheres of the human brain. Davidson initially based his account on case studies of brain-injured individuals. Whereas lesions or tumors in the left frontal lobe appear to be associated with increased risk for depressive episodes, injury to homologous regions in the right frontal lobe appear to be associated with increased risk of manic episodes. Davidson argued that such results are compatible with an hypothesized approach–withdrawal system in which the left frontal region is specialized for approach and the right is specialized for withdrawal. In this account, the left frontal region is said to be involved in the experience of positive emotions such as joy, interest, and happiness. These emotions, in turn, instigate approach behaviors. The right frontal region is said to be involved in the experience of negative emotions such as fear and disgust. The latter emotions, in turn, instigate avoidance behaviors (Davidson, 1992; Schmidt, 1999).

To test this proposal further, Davidson and colleagues presented healthy adults with short film clips designed to elicit either happiness/amusement or disgust. While subjects watched the films, their facial expressions were videotaped and EEG recordings were taken. Results showed that 100% of subjects demonstrated EEG activation patterns consistent with the idea that the left frontal region is specialized for approach and the right is specialized for withdrawal (Davidson, 1992). But these researchers also found considerable individual differences in the degree of asymmetry, which led to a follow-up proposal that people may have stable affective styles. To test the latter proposal, the resting activation of frontal areas in subclinically depressed individuals was compared to that in controls. The researchers found a pattern of right frontal asymmetry in the depressives, which was interpreted to mean there was left frontal underactivation.

Fox and colleagues have also found evidence of stable patterns of emotional reactivity (and asymmetry) in a number of studies of infants and college students (Fox, 1991; Schmidt, 1992). These patterns have also been found to correlate with expected approach–avoidance behavioral strategies such as sociability and shyness.

The Neuroanatomy of Stress and Fear

When adults feel stressed, it is often the case that they have many things to accomplish but not enough time, money, talent, or help to accomplish all of these things. But having too many things to do is only part of the story. The other key factor in stress reactions is fear of punishment (or other negative consequences) for not fulfilling one's responsibilities (e.g., getting fired, getting demoted, paying a late fee, etc.). Given this affinity between fear and stress reactions (McEwen, 1995), these two reactions have been organized together in the present section.

Fear

Much of what we have learned about the neuroanatomy of fear comes from studies of conditioned fear in rats (LeDoux, 1995). Fear can be conditioned by repeatedly presenting a harmless stimulus (e.g., a tone) just before a noxious stimulus occurs (e.g., an electric shock). Over time, the once-neutral stimulus eventually comes to elicit fear in the trained animal.

Through the use of experimental lesioning studies, scientists have found that the key structure in fear conditioning is the amygdala (LeDoux, 1995). The amygdala is an almond-shaped structure located on the inner side of the temporal lobes next to the hippocampus. Information about objects (including their features) arrives at the amygdala by way of pathways originating in the sensory thalamus in the middle of the brain and unimodal association areas in the cortex (e.g., regions of the temporal lobe for auditory stimuli). In addition to associating certain stimuli (e.g., a tone) with fear responses, animals have also been found to associate aspects of their training environment (e.g., their cages) with fear. When components of the hippocampal formation are lesioned, animals retain their conditioned fear of the focal stimulus (e.g., the tone) but lose their conditioned fear of contextual features (e.g., the appearance of their cage). In addition to this double dissociation for context and stimuli, researchers have also found that lesions to the central nucleus of the amygdala produce a reduction in the suppression of the behavior elicited by a fear-inducing stimulus, but no reduction in the tendency to avoid the stimulus. In contrast, animals with lesions in the basolateral region of the amygdala maintained a conditioned suppression but were unable to avoid the stimulus (Killcross, Robbins, & Everitt, 1997).

Further support for the role of the amygdala in negative emotional processing comes from a recent neuroimaging study. Researchers showed that perception of fearful expressions generated greater activity in the amygdala than perception of happy faces (Morris et al., 1996). Moreover, as the intensity of the emotions expressed increased, the disparity in activity for fearful and happy faces increased as well.

After the amygdala receives stimulation from the sensory thalamus and unimodal association cortices, it passes the stimulation onto (1) motor centers responsible for fear behaviors, (2) the vagus nerve to engage fear-related responses in the heart, (3) the spinal cord to engage sympathetic arousal, and (4) the pituitary gland to elicit the release of adrenal hormones which, in turn, precipitate the release of stress hormones (LeDoux, 1995).

Stress

Given the earlier suggestion that there is a connection between fear and stress, it should come as no surprise that the body's reaction to stress involves three of the same structures involved in fear reactions: the amygdala, the hippocampus, and the adrenal glands (McEwen, 1995). However, the construct of stress extends the earlier analysis of fear in several ways. First, prolonged exposure to elevated adrenal steroids has been found to adversely affect the amygdala and the hippocampus (especially the latter). Both of these structures have receptors for stress hormones. Some studies have found that high levels of glucocorticoids may cause atrophy or even death of neurons in the hippocampus. Second, adrenal steroids seem to have a counterregulatory effect in which there is a temporary protection against depletion of important neurotransmitters. To illustrate, animals that have had their adrenal glands removed fall prey to learned helplessness (the animal analog of depression) more quickly than control animals. Third, studies have shown that people react differently to the same stressors. In other words, events that create a great deal of stress for one person may have no effect on another. The key factors that determine individual differences in reactivity to stress include (1) differences in the appraisal process (only the stressed person perceives a threat and lack of control over the threat) and (2) differences in the perceived level of resources available to cope with stressors (McEwen, 1995). When events are perceived as threats and resources are thought to be absent or insufficient, high levels of stress hormones and stress-induced illness ensue.

In a recent neuroimaging study of the effects of stress on memory, researchers found that the following brain areas were activated when victims of a crime (a bank robbery) watched a videotape of the crime: the primary and secondary visual cortex, the posterior cingulate gyrus, and the left orbitofrontal cortex (Fisher, Wik, & Fredrikson, 1996). Decreased blood flow was found in structures such as Broca's area and the left angular gyrus. Given the aforementioned neuroanatomical account of stress, this study should have shown increased levels of activity in the amygdala and hippocampus, but such results did not obtain. Thus, it could be that the amygdala and the hippocampus are active in the early initial processing of a stimulus, but not active during stimulus-based "reliving" or recognition.

The Neuroanatomy and Neurophysiology of Emotional Deficits

Scholars have often debated the wisdom of drawing inferences about normal functioning from abnormal populations (e.g., Kosslyn & Intriligator, 1992). In the present context, neuroscientific studies of several emotional disorders are examined simply to get a sense of brain regions that may participate in normal emotional functioning. In the first line of research to be discussed, the focus is on the possible neuroscientific basis of familial pure depressive disease (FPDD). In the second, the focus is on emotional impairments that arise in Huntington's disease.

Familial Pure Depressive Disease

In the clinical literature, a distinction is often made between unipolar (i.e., "pure") depression and bipolar depression (i.e., manic–depression). Within the unipolar cases, a further distinction is made between familial cases (in which the depression seems to run in families) and nonfamilial cases. In a recent series of imaging studies, scientists have tried to reveal the neuroscientific basis of FPDD using neuroimaging techniques (Drevets & Raichle, 1995).

Results of these studies show that, relative to nondepressed individuals, individuals with FPDD have increased blood flow to three brain areas (the left prefrontal cortex, left amygdala, and left medial thalamus), but decreased blood flow in the ventral medial caudate region of the striatum (Drevets & Raichle, 1995). Further analyses suggested that there appear to be two interconnected circuits implicated in major depression. The first is a limbic–thalamo–cortical (LTC) circuit involving the amygdala, the mediodorsal nucleus of the thalamus, and the ventrolateral and prefrontal cortex. In this circuit, all the connections between regions appear to be excitatory. The second is a limbic–striatal–pallidal–thalamic (LSPT) circuit involving the striatum, ventral pallidum, and most of the regions in the first circuit. Here, the connections between the pallidum and the striatum, and those between the pallidum and thalamus, are said to be inhibitory (Drevets & Raichle, 1995). A related proposal suggests a role for dopaminergic (DA) neurons as well, especially those that project from the substantia nigra and ventral tegmental areas of the midbrain to the striatum, amygdala, and prefrontal cortex. These DA neurons are thought to play an inhibitory role such that a deficiency in DA would be expected to increase activity in the LTC (Drevets & Raichle, 1995).

The foregoing anatomical account suggests that there may be two sources of depression in patients with FPDD. The first would be problems in either the LSPT circuit or the DA projections. If the inhibition imposed by either source is eliminated through damage to these circuits, there might be enhanced activity in the amygdala, striatum, and prefrontal cortex. Increased activity in the amygdala, however, could also be the result of prolonged stress which serves to oversensitize this brain region. Two findings in support of the latter claim are (1) individuals with FPDD who stop taking their antidepressant medicines show abnormal increases in activity in the amygdala and (2) antidepressant medicines substantially decrease blood flow to the amydala (Drevets & Raichle, 1995).

As I noted earlier, Davidson (1992) and Fox (1991) proposed a hemispheric asymmetry model that places less emphasis on subcortical structures such as the amygdala and more emphasis on frontal cortical regions. These researchers have also found individual differences in the degree and stability of hemispheric specialization. In one study, Davidson and colleagues compared the resting activation of frontal areas in subclinically depressed individuals and nondepressed controls. They found a pattern of right frontal asymmetry in the depressives, which was interpreted to mean there was left frontal underactivation.

If this interpretation is correct, however, the results would run somewhat contrary to those reported above in the neuroimaging studies of patients with FPDD. The question then becomes, Why would neuroimaging studies of depression suggest greater activation in the left frontal region while EEG studies suggest lower activation in the left frontal area? Four possible explanations can be proposed. The first is that whereas the neuroimaging studies used patients who were clinically diagnosed with a major depressive disorder (i.e., FPDD), the EEG studies used people who were only mildly depressed. The second explanation is that Davidson and colleagues used the six-site EEG approach. This six-site approach has less spatial resolution than the more precise neuroimaging approaches (see Chapter 1). Perhaps the EEG signals are coming from subcortical areas, then, not from the frontal lobe. The third explanation is that EEG power is assumed to be inversely related to activation, with lower power reflecting greater activation (Lindsley & Wicke, 1974). Davidson and colleagues found higher power readings for the left frontal areas, which they interpreted to mean lower activation. Perhaps the standard interpretation of power is incorrect. At present, it is not clear which of these four explanations is correct. As such, additional research is needed to clarify whether depression results from overactivation of the left frontal region (and other areas like the amygdala) or from underactivation.

Further problems for the left–right asymmetry proposal comes from several recent fMRI and PET studies. In the fMRI study (Teasdale et al., 1999), researchers found that stimuli designed to evoke negative emotions generated increased activity in the right medial and middle frontal gyri, right anterior gingulate gyrus, and right thalamus (consistent with the asymmetry proposal). Stimuli designed to evoke positive emotions, however, produced increased activity in the right and left insula, right inferior frontal gyrus, left splenium, and left precuneus. If the asymmetry proposal is correct, activation should not have been found in these right hemisphere areas. In the PET study (Lane, Reiman, Ahern, Schwartz, & Davidson, 1997), happiness, sadness, and disgust were each associated with increases in activity in the thalamus and Brodmann Area 9 of the prefrontal cortex, as well as with anterior and temporal structures. Thus, in both studies, a strict left–frontal–positive/right–frontal–negative dissociation did not occur. It is also curious that the amygdala was not found to be especially active in either study, given that other neuro-imaging studies (e.g., Schneider et al., 1997) found increased activity in the left amygdala for positive and negative emotions.

Perhaps the discrepant findings for hemispheric asymmetry derive from the fact that the authors did not equate stimuli for degree of arousal. When Canli, Desmond, Zhao, Glover, and Gabrieli (1998) did so in their neuroimaging study of 12 women, they found that overall activity was lateralized to the left hemisphere for positive emotions and toward the right hemisphere for negative emotions. Other reasons for discrepant results pertain to the fact that (1) some researchers only used one gender (females) while others used both genders; (2) some used PET while others used fMRI or EEG methods; (3) some assessed resting levels of activity in the absence of stimuli while others presented emotional stimuli; and (4) some asked participants to generate emotional feelings from memory while others presented emotional stimuli to subjects.

Huntington's Disease

Huntington's disease is an autosomal dominant disorder of the brain that includes clinical features such as chorea (spasms), mood change, cognitive impairments, and dementia (Zakzanis, 1998). The most pronounced cognitive deficits are problems in delayed recall, cognitive flexibility, and manual dexterity. The primary site of cell loss in patients with Huntington's disease occurs in the striatum portion of the basal ganglia. This cell loss, in turn, produces two main changes in the level of neurotransmitters in the brain (Folstein, 1989). First, inhibitory GABA-ergic neurons that project to the pallidum are lost, resulting in decreases in GABA. Second, receptors for DA in striatal cells are lost, resulting in increases in DA (because the DA does not bind to these sites). Both of these changes together lead to the expectation of increased neuronal activity in the LCT circuit (due to loss of inhibitory forces on this circuit) and increased depression in patients with Huntington's disease (Drevets & Raichle, 1995). Studies, in fact, show that patients with Huntington's disease are four to 10 times more likely to experience depression than other patients with disabling conditions (Drevets & Raichle, 1995).

Another curious and disturbing finding that recently emerged in studies of patients with Huntington's disease is that these individuals show deficits in recognizing facial expressions of anger and fear, and are particularly poor at recognizing facial expressions of disgust (Sprengelmeyer et al., 1996). Such findings are consistent with the results of studies of individuals who have bilateral lesions of the amygdala. These individuals also show impaired recognition of fear and anger when stimuli are presented in either the visual or the auditory modalities (Scott et al., 1997). These findings together suggest that the basal ganglia and associated structures (e.g., the amygdala) may be important for recognizing the negative emotions.

CONCLUSIONS, CAVEATS, AND INSTRUCTIONAL IMPLICATIONS

Comparison of the psychological and neuroscientific perspectives on emotion reveals that these two traditions have apparently not influenced each other to a great extent. For example, the psychological "carving" of emotion into specific components (e.g., appraisal, etc.) has not led to the systematic discovery of specific regions of the brain that are uniquely dedicated to carrying out one and only one of these components. In a related way, the findings of recent neuroimaging and gross electrical recording studies have generally not led to significant changes in contemporary psychological models of emotion.

This apparent lack of overlap in the two perspectives could be explained in three ways. First, researchers in these traditions have not always been interested in asking the same questions. Note how the psychological question "How might the emotion of joy be distinguished from the emotion of pride?" is different than the neuroscientific question "Which regions of the brain seem to be important for emotional responding?" Second, whereas psychological approaches have tended to focus on multiple emotions, neuroscientific approaches have tended to focus on single emotions. Third, different species have been used in the two traditions (e.g., humans vs. rats). These three problems are further complicated by the fact that in certain cases (e.g., depression), the results of several neuroscientific experiments conflict (e.g., the left frontal lobe is overactivated vs. underactivated). The findings as a whole have even led some scholars to wonder whether there really are emotion-specific brain structures (Davidson & Ekman, 1994).

Thus, it seems safe to say that there is still much to learn about the nature of emotion and its implementation in the human brain. Two lines of research would seem to be particularly important in the future. In the first, neuroscientists should use the emerging psychological consensus regarding the nature of emotion as a guide to see if there are regions of the brain that correspond to the common components that have been alleged in the psychological models. In the second line of research, neuroscientists should conduct a number of replication studies in which individuals of the same species, age, and background are placed within the same methodological conditions (e.g., presentation of the same stimuli and use of the same kind of neuroimaging technique). It is important to determine whether conflicting findings reflect the "unlocalized" nature of emotions or differences in methodologies.

As for instructional implications, it should be recalled that neuroscientific research should be viewed as relevant to education to the extent that it (1) helps corroborate existing psychological models of learning, cognitive development, or motivation; or (2) explains recurrent findings from psychological experiments (see Chapters 1 and 8). Given the lack of overlap between these traditions in the case of emotions (see above), it might be said that the available neuroscientific work on emotions is largely irrelevant to the field of education. As I noted earlier, however, there are a few ways that neuroscientific evidence might ultimately lead to new insights into learning after additional studies are conducted. First, there are findings in the area of memory that could have emotional underpinnings. For example, there is the phenomenon of flashbulb memory. At present, scientists still do not know why people have better memories for upsetting events than for neutral events. It could be that high levels of emotional arousal help in the consolidation of memories. The amygdala is, after all, adjacent to the hippocampus in the brain, and the hippocampus has been found to be important to the consolidation of memories (see Chapter 3). Or, perhaps, memory is enhanced because emotions engage an orienting reflex and increased attention (Porges, 1995). It could also be the case that emotional feelings are simply contextual cues (like any other aspect of a situation) that can be used to help retrieve memories (Anderson, 1995). The latter explanation is consistent with the findings from mood-congruency experiments in which people who are induced to feel a certain way when learning material (e.g., sad) recall more when they are induced to feel the same way during the test situation (e.g., sad) than when they are induced to feel a different way (e.g., happy). Either way, it should be clear that instruction is more likely to be effective if it can somehow enlist the help of student emotions. As I noted earlier, emotions determine the goals students set, the things they attend to, and their depth of processing.

A second way that emotional research could be viewed as relevant to education concerns the centrality of emotions in the human motivational system (Pintrich & Schunk, 1996). Attribution theories (e.g.,

Weiner, 1985) have shown how people report feeling different emotions when they attribute outcomes to different kinds of antecedent causes. For example, students who get low scores on a test and blame their teachers for making the test too hard might feel anger at their teachers rather than embarrassment or disappointment with themselves. In contrast, students who attribute the failure to their lack of skill or lack of studying would probably feel different emotions. In the proactive sense, anticipated outcomes that are based on attributions, expectations, and values (Wigfield & Eccles, 1992) can lead a student to make choices in school (e.g., try hard vs. not try hard; choose major X vs. choose major Y). Of course, there is more to motivation than emotions (e.g., self-efficacy, values, etc.). Psychological work on these other aspects of motivation were not described in this chapter because neuroscientists have not examined these issues. In the present author's view, neuroscientific work on interest would be a useful new way to extend what has already been done in the area of motivation. Interest has been alleged to be a basic emotion with neural underpinnings by emotion researchers (e.g., Porges, 1995) and also a core aspect of motivation (Wigfield & Eccles, 1992). Moreover, it would be fascinating to learn that students may be born with certain interests (e.g., reading vs. math) that affect their decision to pursue certain subjects and to avoid others. Many have found that early readers have an unusual and early interest in books (see Chapter 6). Such findings would not negate, of course, the ample evidence that many interests are acquired through experience and socialization (Wigfield & Eccles, 1992).

A final way that neuroscientifically oriented research could have relevance to education derives from recent arguments made by evolutionary psychologists (Geary, 1998; Pinker, 1997). Evolutionary psychologists have noted that the size of brain regions that are devoted to particular kinds of processing (e.g., visual) differ by species. Such differences, in turn, correlate with the environmental demands placed on animals of these species. For example, an unusually large portion of the primate cortex is devoted to visual processing. Analysis of the feeding, sleeping, and mating habits of primates reveals that they need a considerable amount of visual processing skill to survive. Using similar arguments, evolutionary psychologists have proposed that humans are born with brain systems that help them develop sophisticated naive theories of physics, biology, and psychology. These theories, in turn, bias the way children learn content in these domains and also explain an inherent sociability and need for affiliation in the human species. At present, however, researchers have yet to find brain regions that are devoted to these three naive theories. Should this account prove to be true, it could have many implications for issues of instructional content (what to teach), timing (when to teach), and approach (solitary work vs. cooperative collaboration). It could also be part of the explanation as to why children perform better in school when they view their teachers as caring (Wentzel, 1997). Regardless, the evolutionary account requires further study.

CHAPTER 6

Reading

The ability to read is arguably the most important skill that children can acquire. Proficient readers not only do well in school, they also gain massive amounts of knowledge across their lifetimes. Poor readers, in contrast, have a great deal of difficulty in school and often end up in low-wage jobs or in correctional institutions. The significance of reading in people's lives could well explain why the scientific literature on reading is enormous and extends back to the late 19th century.

For obvious reasons, then, it would not be possible to review all aspects of the literature on reading in a single chapter. One could, however, review just those aspects that are germane to the central issues of this book (e.g., the compatibility of the psychological and neuroscientific perspectives on reading). The first two sections of this chapter describe the psychological and neuroscientific perspectives on reading, respectively. In the third section, I focus on the compatibility of these two perspectives as well as the instructional implications of an integrated view of reading.

PSYCHOLOGICAL PERSPECTIVES ON READING

My goal in the present section is to provide insight into the essential nature of reading ability. To this end, I shall first examine a popular model of reading that captures most of the core operations that have been proposed by psychologists over the years (i.e., the Seidenberg and McClelland model). Next, I shall extend this model somewhat by considering what people do when they try to comprehend lengthy passages. In the final section, I devote attention to psychological studies that have revealed the key behavioral differences between good readers and poor readers.

The Seidenberg and McClelland Model of Reading

In 1989, Mark Seidenberg and James McClelland proposed a model of reading that currently has many adherents (Adams, 1990; Pressley, 1997). In what follows, this model is described to give a sense of how contemporary psychologists decompose reading into its component operations. The central idea is that skilled readers interpret text by way of four interactive processors that operate in their minds (see Figure 6.1; Seidenberg & McClelland, 1989). Let's examine each of these processors in turn.

The Orthographic Processor

Writers encode their ideas in strings of orthographic symbols (e.g., English letters, Chinese characters, etc.) and hope that people will get their message. For example, an English-speaking man might jot down the string of letters "I'm at the store. Be home by 3" in a note to his wife. Clearly, the wife could not decipher this note if she lacked the ability to recognize her husband's pen marks as legal instances of English letters and words. Imagine what would happen if her husband's handwriting were particularly bad or if she could only recognize Chinese characters. According to Seidenberg and McClelland (1989), the ability to recognize legal instances of text is made possible by the orthographic processor shown in Figure 6.1. It can be thought of as a storehouse of orthographic knowledge.

The orthographic processor is said to contain a large quantity of interconnected "units" that are thought to bear a close correspondence to neural assemblies. Each unit is responsible for recognizing parts of letters, whole letters, or whole words. Associations form between the units

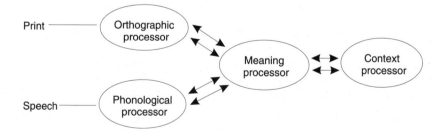

FIGURE 6.1. The four processors of the reading system. After Seidenberg and McClelland (1989).

for letters when certain letters (e.g., "q") frequently co-occur with other letters (e.g., "u") in the texts that people read. Any familiar word, then, is really a highly associated pattern of letters, and each letter in the word "primes" the perception of the others. As a result, the entire word is recognized very quickly and automatically.

Letter associations also help skilled readers do three other things. First, associations help readers process the proper order of letters in a word. For example, although both of the two strings THE and HTE have the letters needed for the word "the," only the former would be recognized as such. Second, associations help skilled readers perceive pseudowords. *Pseudowords* are letter strings that involve high-frequency associations but are not real words (e.g., "mave" and "teel"). Third, associations help a skilled reader divide a word into syllables. For example, whereas "dr" is an acceptable combination of letters that maps onto the sounds of spoken English, "dn" is not. As a result, a skilled reader who encounters the word "midnight" would visually divide this word into "mid" and "night." In contrast, skilled readers would not visually divide "address" into "add" and "ress." Moreover, a skilled reader implicitly knows that vowels seem to pull their adjacent consonants into a cluster of association patterns. For example, the first "a" in "partial" pulls the "p" and "r" toward itself. This fact combined with the fact that "rt" is an unacceptable spoken combination means that "partial" would be divided into "par" and "tial" (Adams, 1990).

It is interesting to note that, historically, written language did not use spacing and punctuation to delineate words (Just & Carpenter, 1987). As a result, readers had to rely exclusively on their orthographic knowledge to make sense of a sentence. To see how this might work, note that you *can* read the following sentence even though there are no spaces between the words:

THATWASDELICIOUS

The Meaning Processor

Of course, comprehending a sentence requires far more than the ability to determine whether letter strings are orthographically acceptable or familiar. For example, the sentence "Trat distle quas" contains three acceptable combinations of letters (according to frequency), but it is meaningless. Similarly, the sentence "The octogenarian insinuated himself into our organization" would be meaningless to someone who knows she has seen the letter strings "octogenarian" and "insinuated" before, but cannot remember what these words mean. Thus, sentence comprehension requires both an orthographic processor to recognize letter strings and a meaning processor to access word meanings.

Two views have been proposed regarding how meanings are assigned to words. According to the *lexical access* view, entire word meanings are stored in a person's mental *lexicon*. The lexicon is simply a "dictionary" in your memory that organizes word meanings in terms of lists of attributes, or schemata. When a written word is perceived, its meanings are accessed if the resting activation levels of these word meanings in memory are high enough (Just & Carpenter, 1987; see Chapter 3 for more on the construct of resting activation). Moreover, the higher the resting activation level, the faster a word meaning will be retrieved. Word meanings attain a high activation level if the words to which they are attached occur frequently. Thus, the meanings of frequent words are accessed faster than the meanings of infrequent words.

The second view derives from recent *connectionist* theories. According to this view, word meanings are represented in the meaning processor as associated sets of primitive meaning elements, in the same way that spellings of familiar words are represented in the orthographic processor as associated sets of letters and letter parts (Adams, 1990). A person's experience determines which meaning elements get associated and stored for a given word (Hintzman, 1986). For example, a child who hears the word "dog" applied to a specific dog in a specific context might associate the whole experience with the word "dog." The next time she hears the word "dog" applied, however, it might be with a different dog in a different context. According to the connectionist view, those aspects of the second context that are similar to aspects of the first context (e.g., both dogs had a flea collar) would become associated and stored with the word "dog." Over time, a consistent set of meaning elements would be distilled from these repeated encounters with dogs. Each element would be highly associated with the others, and would therefore "prime" one's memory for the others. Moreover, some aspects of the meaning of "dog" would be more central to its meaning and reflect consistent correlations of attributes (e.g., "has fur" and "barks"). Such attributes would be accessed the fastest when the single word "dog" is read. Other meaning elements that are somewhat less central (e.g., "has a flea collar") would also be accessible but would be accessed more slowly if at all when the word is read in isolation.

As Figure 6.1 shows, the meaning processor is directly linked to the orthographic processor. This depiction means that the output of each processor can help the other do its job better. In support of this claim, Whittlesea and Cantwell (1987) found that when pseudowords are given a meaningful definition, subjects perceived these words faster than when such words lacked a definition. This improved perceptibility lasted for at least 24 hours after meaning instruction, even when subjects could not recall the supplied meaning later on. Thus, the meaning processor helped the orthographic processor do its job better. Perhaps more importantly, the arrows between the two processors suggest that associations form between orthographic units and meaning units. In this way, the sight of the words can and should activate meanings automatically.

The Phonological Processor

As was the case for the orthographic and meaning processors, the phonological processor is said to consist of units that form associations with each other. Phonological units correspond to *phonemes* in the reader's spoken language. Phonemes such as "buh," "ah," and "tuh" can be combined into syllables such as "ba-" and "-at", and also into words such as "bat." The auditory representation of a word, syllable, or phoneme is comprised by an activated set of specific units in the phonological processor (Adams, 1990).

When skilled readers see a written word, they do not have to translate it phonologically in order for its meaning to be accessed. Many studies have shown that meaning can be accessed simply by a visual pattern of letters (Adams, 1990; Seidenberg & McClelland, 1989). And yet, skilled readers often *do* translate words phonologically when they read.

Why would people perform some operation when they do not have to? The answer seems to be that the phonological processor provides a certain degree of redundancy with the information provided by the other processors. This redundancy can be quite helpful when the information provided by the other processors is incomplete, deceptive, or weakly specified (Stanovich, 1980; Adams, 1990).

More specifically, the phonological processor seems to provide two important services to the overall reading system. First, it provides an alphabetic backup system that may be crucial for maintaining fast and accurate reading (Adams, 1990). This backup system exists mainly because the orthography of written English largely obeys the *alphabetic principle*: written symbols (i.e., graphemes) correspond to spoken sounds (i.e., phonemes). Although this grapheme–phoneme correspondence is not one-to-one or perfectly regular, it is nevertheless sufficiently predictable to be useful (Just & Carpenter, 1987). As a result, the phonological processor could provide helpful information in a variety of situations. For example, consider the case in which a reader knows the meaning of a spoken word but has never seen it written down. There would be no direct connection between (1) the units corresponding to the letters of this word in the orthographic processor and (2) the units corresponding to the meaning of this word in the meaning processor. There would, however, be a connection between the phonological processor units and the meaning processor units for this word. If the word obeys the alphabetic principle fairly well, the person would be able to "sound it out" and hear him- or herself saying the familiar word. This pronunciation would then access the meaning of the word. Over repeated readings, the two-way association between the phonological processor units and the meaning processor units for this word would become a three-way association between the orthographic, meaning, and phonological units.

The second service provided by the phonological processor has to do with a reader's memory for what he or she has just read. In Chapter 3, we learned that psychologists believe that there is a phonological loop in working memory that is used to rehearse and maintain information for later processing (Baddeley, 1999). When people read, they have to take all of the words in a sentence and put them together into a meaningful whole (Just & Carpenter, 1987). This integration requires working memory because when someone reads from left to right, only one or two words fall within that person's visual fixation span. That is, all of the words to the left of a visual fixation point must be retained in working memory.

The Context Processor

The context processor has the job of constructing an on-line, coherent interpretation of text (Adams, 1990). The output of this processor is a mental representation of everything that a reader has read so far. For example, when one reads the sentence "When the president came in, all of the reporters rose," the context accessed may be a mental image of the President of the United States walking up to the podium in the White House press room. Whereas some researchers (e.g., Just & Carpenter, 1987) call this image a *referential representation* of the text, others (e.g. van Dijk & Kintsch, 1983) call it a *situation model*. For simplicity, we can use the latter term here.

Semantic, pragmatic, and syntactic knowledge all contribute to the construction of a situation model (Seidenberg & McClelland, 1989). For example, when skilled readers encounter the sentence "John went to the store to buy a _____," they use their semantic knowledge to access the meanings of all of the words in this sentence. In addition, they use their pragmatic knowledge to figure out that "John" will buy something that people usually buy at stores. If the blank was filled in by "savings bond," readers would likely be surprised when their eyes reached the word "savings."

Syntactic knowledge also prompts the reader to form certain expectations about what will occur next (Garrett, 1990; Just & Carpenter, 1987). To see how the syntactic "parser" operates, we need to draw on linguists' notions of grammatical rules. Many linguists argue that there are certain *types* of sentences and each type can be produced using a specific set of rules (Lasnick, 1990). For example, each of the following sentences can be produced by using the same three rules:

- The fat boy hit the round ball.
- The girl chewed an apple.
- A man drew a picture.

These rules are:

Rule 1   Sentence = Noun Phrase + Verb Phrase (i.e., S→NP + VP)
Rule 2   Verb Phrase = Verb + Noun Phrase (i.e., VP→V + NP)
Rule 3   Noun Phrase = Determiner + (optional adjective) + Noun (i.e., NP →Det + (adj)+ N)

Linguists believe that given a specific input sentence and its knowledge of grammatical rules, the human mind builds up mental representation of the sentence, component by component. For example, upon reading the word "the," the rule for producing noun phrases is elicited. Implicitly, the mind says, "OK. A noun phrase must be starting." Given that a determiner has already been encountered, Rule 3 (above) sets up the expectation that either an adjective or a noun will be encountered next. When the word "fat" is read in sentence 1 above, it is assigned the slot for adjective. Having organized the words "the" and "fat" together, Rule 3 now sets up the expectation that the next word will likely be a noun, and so on. In order for this system to work, written words (e.g., "fat") have to be mentally associated with grammatical classes (e.g., "adjective"). Thus, the model so far suggests that words have associated spellings, meanings, pronunciations, and grammatical classes.

The model of proficient reading in Figure 6.1 shows the two-way relationship between the context processor and the meaning processor. The arrows imply that the prior context can influence the meaning assigned to a word and that current meanings influence the construction of a situation model. Thus, when skilled readers process the sentence "John removed the thorn from the rose," they assign a different meaning to "rose" than they would if they read the sentence "At the baseball game, the crowd rose to sing the national anthem." Thus, the model suggests that expectations derive from the meaning of words and the grammatical category assigned to a word.

But research has shown that the context–meaning effects are weak relative to the orthography–meaning effects. That is, readers are much better at predicting possible meanings of a word based on its perceived spelling than they are at predicting which word will follow a preceding context (Adams, 1990). When context–meaning links conflict with orthography–meaning links, the latter win out. Thus, skilled reading consists, first and foremost, of learning the correspondences between written words and their meanings. Context effects occur *after* words are perceived and various possible meanings are accessed. In general, however, context, orthography, meanings, and phonology all work in concert to help a reader construct the best possible interpretation of a text.

Further Explorations into the Nature of Reading Comprehension

Although the Seidenberg and McClelland model is useful for providing a good overall sense of skilled reading, it fails to address several important issues in the area of reading comprehension. In the present section, these issues will be discussed more fully. In the first part, I consider important aspects of reading comprehension that derive from a reader's knowledge (structural aspects). Then, I consider aspects that derive from a reader's strategic behaviors (functional aspects).

Structural Aspects of Comprehension

Researchers who study reading comprehension have relied heavily on the construct of *schema* (plural, *schemata*). A *schema* is a mental representation of what multiple instances of something have in common. For example, a schema for a house specifies the things that most houses have in common. Besides having schemata for things like houses, skilled readers and writers are thought to have schemata for specific types of texts, too. The two main schemata for texts that have been examined extensively are those for *narrative* and *expository* texts. In what follows, we shall see how schemata for specific topics (e.g., houses), narratives, and expository texts help students comprehend and remember what they are reading.

When readers have schematized knowledge for things (e.g., houses) and events (e.g., funerals), they are better able to assimilate the information presented in some text than when they lack such knowledge. For example, readers who have never attended a funeral would have more trouble comprehending sentences such as "Mary straightened her black dress as she walked closer to express her condolences" than readers who have attended many funerals. In fact, experienced readers would not even need the writer to explicitly say that Mary was at a funeral (they would guess that she was). Comprehension is all about understanding what is going on in a passage. Schemata for topics help a reader figure out what is going on (e.g., where the character is, what he or she is doing and why, etc.).

Turning next to other kinds of schemata, note that some texts take on the structure of a narrative (e.g., stories) while others take on a more expository structure (e.g., textbooks). The structural characteristics of most narratives include the fact that there are (1) *characters* who have goals and motives for performing actions; (2) *temporal* and *spatial placements* in which the story takes place; (3) *complications* and *major goals* of main characters; (4) *plots* and *resolutions* of complications; (5) *affect patterns* (i.e., emotional and other responses to the story line); (6) *points*, *morals*, and *themes*; and (7) *points of view* and *perspectives* (Graesser, Golding, & Long, 1991).

A person who writes a narrative, then, has schematized knowledge of the above components of a story and tries to "fill in" the components as he or she writes. An author does so with the expectation that his or her readers also have this schematized knowledge. As each part of a story unfolds, readers rely on their narrative schemata to form expectations as to what will come next. Skilled writers play off these expectations to occasionally surprise readers or "leave them hanging" (as cliff-hangers do). Moreover, readers use their schemata for narratives to help them judge whether or not a story is a good one and also to create a situation model of what they have read.

Whereas the main goal of a narrative text (e.g., "Snow White") is to tell a story to entertain readers, the main goal of an expository text (e.g., a textbook) is to provide information so that the reader can learn something (Weaver & Kintsch, 1991). Consequently, schemata for expository texts differ from those for narratives. The two most cited theoretical models of expository schemata are those of Meyer (1985) and Kintsch (1982). In Kintsch's (1982) model, three main relations make up the schemata for expository texts:

1. *General–particular* relations, which have to do with identifying, defining, classifying, or illustrating things (e.g., "An igneous rock is a rock that. . . ").
2. *Object–object* relations, which have to do with comparing or

contrasting things (e.g., "Evergreen trees differ from deciduous trees in that . . . ").

3. *Object–part* relations, which have to do with causal relations, the arrangements of parts in an object, or how the parts work (e.g., "The carburetor in an engine has the job of . . . ").

In Meyer's (1985) model, the ideas in a passage are also said to stand in certain relations to each other. Analyses of many common expository texts show that writers arrange their ideas into five common relations:

1. *Collection*: a relation that shows how things are related together into a group (e.g., "There are seven types of vehicles on the road today. First, there are . . . ").
2. *Causation*: a relation that shows how one event is the antecedent cause of another event (e.g., "The tanker spilled all of its oil into the sea. As a result, the sea life . . . ").
3. *Response*: a relation that shows how one idea is a problem and another is a solution to the problem (e.g., "A significant number of homeless people have a substance abuse problem. It should be clear that homelessness will not diminish until increased money goes to treatment of this disorder . . . ").
4. *Comparison*: a relation in which the similarities and differences between things are pointed out (e.g., "Piaget and Vygotsky both emphasized egocentric speech; however, Vygotsky viewed it more as . . . ").
5. *Description*: a relation in which more information about something is given, such as attributes, specifics, manners, or settings (e.g., "Newer oil tankers are safer than they used to be. These days they have power steering and double hulls.").

Because these relations pertain to how the ideas are arranged in some text, they are said make up the "prose structure" of the text. Writers hope that the arrangement of ideas in their readers' minds is the same as the arrangement of ideas in the text.

A person who writes an expository textbook, then, has schematized knowledge of the relations identified by Kintsch (1982) and Meyer (1985) and also knows the conventional ways of communicating these relations. The most common way to prompt readers to recognize a particular relation is to place sentences close together. When one sentence follows another, skilled readers try to form a connection between them. If a writer fears that his or her readers will not make the connection even when sentences are placed in close proximity, he or she can use various *signaling* devices to make the connection explicit. For example, to convey Meyer's (1985) comparison relation, a writer might use the words "In contrast, . . . " To signal causal relations, he or she might use the words "As a result, . . . "

In addition to helping readers form expectations, knowledge of prose structure also helps readers comprehend and retain more of what they read (Meyer, 1985; Weaver & Kintsch, 1991). In particular, the five relations identified by Meyer often serve as an author's main point or thesis. Main ideas are connected by one of these five relations and lesser ideas are subsumed beneath this overall relation. People who first encode the main point and then attach additional ideas to the main point demonstrate better comprehension and memory of the ideas in a passage than people who treat paragraphs as a string of individual ideas.

Functional Aspects of Comprehension

In addition to having structural knowledge of topics and the various kinds of texts (e.g., narrative vs. expository), readers also need to engage in a variety of on-line processes in order to enhance their reading comprehension (Paris, Wasik, & Turner, 1991; Pressley et al., 1994). These processes are collectively called "reading strategies" and include: (1) goal setting, (2) inference making, (3) identifying the main idea, (4) summarizing, (5) predicting, (6) monitoring, and (7) backtracking.

Setting a goal for reading is the first thing that readers need to do before they read (Pressley et al., 1994). Reading is a purposeful activity in that we read things for different reasons (Paris et al., 1991). For example, whereas we usually read a newspaper to find out what is happening in the world, we read spy novels simply to be entertained or to take our minds off work. Similarly, sometimes we only want a rough sense of what an author is trying to say, so we only skim the pages for major points. Other times we really want to process everything an author says, so we read every line very carefully (e.g., when students read a textbook right before a test). Goal setting is crucial because the goals we set can either enhance or limit what we get from reading. For example, if someone sets the goal of "pronouncing all of the words correctly" but fails to set the goal of "learning something," he or she is unlikely to engage in any of the remaining strategies.

Inference making is, perhaps, the most widely studied reading strategy (Paris et al., 1991). Readers make inferences in order to (1) elaborate on the meaning of an individual sentence and (2) integrate the meanings of several sentences in a text (Alba & Hasher, 1982). For example, when readers encounter sentences such as "The man stirred his coffee," many of them elaborate on the ideas presented by inferring that he used a spoon. In addition, when presented with a pair of sentences such as

"Joe smoked four packs a day.
After he died, his wife sold her Phillip Morris stocks,"

many readers would infer that smoking caused Joe to die. Thus, the two ideas of smoking and dying are integrated together through a causal relation. Moreover, inferences play an important role in the reader's construction of a situation model for the text he or she is reading. As I mentioned above, the principle source of inferences is a reader's schematized knowledge of topics such as "coffee" and "cigarettes."

Why do readers make inferences when they read? It seems that a reader's mind is always trying to make sense of what it is encountering. One way of making sense of things is to make the information presented more concrete and specific. So, when people read the sentence above about stirring, their minds naturally ask questions such as "What kind of thing do people usually use to stir their coffee?" Notice that the inference that a spoon was used is merely probabilistic. People sometimes use whatever is handy, such as the handle of a fork.

As to why we make intersentence inferences, it is helpful to repeat a point made earlier: it seems that the mind is always asking "How does this new sentence relate to the sentences that I already read?" When two events co-occur close in time, it is natural to think that the prior one caused the later one (Bullock, Gelman, & Baillargeon, 1982). For example, because the first sentence above is about smoking and the second one right after it is about dying, it is natural to assume that smoking killed Joe. Similarly, if one reads "The floor was just mopped. I fell," it is natural to assume that the speaker slipped on the floor. It is possible, however, that smoking did not kill Joe and that the person fell because of something else (e.g., tripping over a bucket). Thus, once again we see that inferences are not necessary conclusions, they are merely probabilistic guesses.

In addition to causal connections, there are a variety of other intersentence connections that could be made. For example, readers naturally link up a pronoun in a second sentence to a person's name in a first sentence (e.g., "Mary saw the doctor. She said . . ."). Similar to causal inferences, inferences about pronouns are also probabilistic (i.e., "she" could be a female doctor).

Besides inference making, a second important comprehension strategy is *identifying the main idea*. In order to identify the main idea of some passage, readers need to assess the relevance of each idea and then rank-order ideas in terms of centrality or importance (van Dijk & Kintsch, 1983). As I noted above, people often rely on the prose structure of some passage to identify the main idea. In addition, they have also been found to use various signals in the text.

Besides being central to comprehension, an additional reason why identifying the main idea is an important strategy is that it is a prerequisite skill for performing the third important reading strategy: *summarizing*. In order to create a summary, you need to be able to delete unimportant ideas and retain just the "gist" of what is written. The gist, in turn, is comprised mostly of the main ideas.

The fourth important reading strategy is *predicting*. Predicting consists simply of forming expectations regarding what will happen next in a narrative story or anticipating what the author of an expository text will say next. Good writers are skilled at helping readers make predictions and also good at violating expectations in such a way that it is entertaining.

The fifth reading strategy is called *comprehension monitoring*. Simply put, comprehension monitoring is the ability to "know when you don't know," that is, it is the ability to detect a comprehension failure (Markman, 1981). As I suggested earlier, reading does not consist of simply knowing how to sound out words. Rather, it consists of extracting meaning from texts. If a portion of a text does not make sense, readers should recognize that the main goal of reading (i.e., extracting meaning) has not been met.

When readers recognize that something that they just read does not make sense, they have two options: (1) they could say, "Oh well! Let's just read on!," or (2) they could decide to do something about their comprehension failure. The latter option brings us to our sixth and final strategy, *backtracking*. Backtracking consists of rereading a portion of a text when a comprehension failure occurs. Garner (1987) suggests that readers backtrack in response to four judgments and beliefs:

1. They do not understand or remember what they just read.
2. They believe that they can find the information needed to resolve the difficulty in the text.
3. The prior material must be scanned to locate the helpful information.
4. Information from several prior sentences may need to be combined and manipulated to resolve the comprehension problem.

Individual Differences in Reading Skills

In any given grade in school, there are children who are below average in their reading ability, children who read at grade level, and children who are above average. As one final way to gain insight into the nature of reading, we can consider how children in the first and third groups have been found to differ from each other.

By way of introduction, it is important to note that there are a number of ways in which good readers could differ from poor readers. On the one hand, they could differ in terms of general factors such as intelligence, working memory capacity, perceptual ability, rule induction, and metacognition. On the other hand, they could differ in terms of reading-specific processes such as word recognition, use of context, phonemic awareness, and comprehension strategies. It turns out that significant differences have been found between good and poor readers for all of these variables (Stanovich, 1980, 1986, 1988a). The question is, however, which of these variables seem to most clearly distinguish good readers from poor readers.

Careful reviews of the literature have revealed three particularly important differences between good and poor readers. First, good readers are better than poor readers at recognizing words automatically. When word recognition is automatic, a reader can focus his or her attention on higher level sentence integration and semantic processing (see Chapter 4 for more on attention). However, automatic recognition is most important in the first and second grades because most high-frequency words are automatized to adult levels by the time the average child reaches the third grade (Stanovich, 1980). Beginning in the third grade, the second and most important difference between good and poor readers emerges: good readers are able to *rapidly* recognize words and subword units. Speed is important because, as I noted earlier, readers need to be able to operate on information in working memory before it dissipates. The third important difference between good and poor readers concerns the ability to recode print items into a phonological representation. As I noted earlier, phonological recoding facilitates reading by (1) providing a redundant pathway for accessing word meaning and (2) providing a more stable code for the information that is held in working memory (Adams, 1990; Stanovich, 1980).

At one time, the ability to use prior context was also thought to be a major difference between good and poor readers. After many years of research, however, this proposal turns out to be incorrect. In fact, poor readers use prior context as much if not more than good readers and are likely to make many substitution errors when they encounter an unfamiliar word (Adams, 1990; Stanovich, 1988a). Skilled readers rely much more heavily on direct connections between orthography and meaning than on context. Context only exerts an experimental effect on good readers when the text is artificially doctored or degraded. Thus, whereas good readers rely on context less and less as they get older, poor readers do not show a similar kind of decreasing reliance on context, presumably because they have so much trouble recognizing and deciphering a word. Of course, this is not to say that context is irrelevant to good readers. As I mentioned earlier, context serves as an important backup system to the connections between text and meanings.

Why are good readers better at automatic and fast recognition and pronunciation of words than poor readers? From what we know about the nature of skill acquisition and the formation of associations (Anderson, 1990), it seems clear that good readers have had considerably more practice at recognizing and pronouncing words than have poor readers. A likely cause of practice differences could be the fact that children are grouped by reading ability starting in the first grade. Children in higher groups are given more opportunities for practice than children in lower groups and the initial gap between groups widens with age (Stanovich, 1986). But there may also be neurological and other differences between good readers and poor readers that may limit the extent to which practice seems to be effective. In the next section, we shall consider this neurological possibility and other related issues.

NEUROSCIENTIFIC PERSPECTIVES ON READING

In the previous section, we saw that the psychological description of reading refers to three main hypothetical constructs: processors, schemata, and strategies. In the present section, we shall examine the conceptualization of reading that has emerged from the neuroscientific literature and also consider the similarities between the former and latter descriptions. The discussion proceeds as follows. First, I provide an overview of the neuroscientific literature. Then, I consider the neurological basis of reading disability. Finally, I address the issue of whether there is a neuroscientific basis to phenomena such as reading readiness and precocious reading.

Overview of the Neuroscientific Approach

Inasmuch as animals cannot read, cognitive neuroscientists have had to rely exclusively on data from neuroimaging studies and studies of brain-injured adults to infer the component skills of reading. Thus, the neuro-science of reading is likely to be fundamentally different than the neuro-science of brain development, memory and attention (which have relied on data from animal studies).

Studies of brain-injured adults have revealed a number of distinct (but sometimes co-occurring) deficits. At one time, the typical approach was to classify collections of deficits in terms of syndromes (e.g., dyslexia with dysgraphia vs. dyslexia without dysgraphia). Since the 1960s, information-processing and other psychological accounts have prompted investigators to subdivide acquired reading problems into two general classes: (1) those related to visually analyzing the attributes of written words (*visual word-form dyslexias*) and (2) those related to pre-sumed later stages of the reading process (*central dyslexias*) (McCarthy & Warrington, 1990).

Visual word-form dyslexias include spelling dyslexia, neglect dys-lexia, and attentional dyslexia (McCarthy & Warrington, 1990). *Spell-ing dyslexia* is manifested in brain-injured adults who read letter by let-ter (e.g., when they see "dog" they say "D, O, G spells 'dog'"). Such patients may have normal spelling and writing ability, but they cannot read back what they have written down. The tendency to spell is a strat-egy that patients seem to use to overcompensate for an inability to recognize words as units. In most cases, spelling dyslexics have lesions located near the junctions of the occipital, temporal, and parietal lobes (the left angular gyrus). *Neglect dyslexia* consists of omitting or misread-ing the initial or terminal parts of words (e.g., they see "his" when confronted with "this," "wet" when confronted with "let," "together" when confronted with "whether"). Case studies reveal that whereas the left (initial) portion of words is neglected when there is damage to the right parietal lobe, the right (terminal) part of words is neglected when there is damage to the left parietal lobe. *Attentional dyslexics* can read individual letters quite well (e.g., "A"), but have significantly more diffi-culty when they have to read individual letters that are flanked by other letters in the visual field (e.g., the "A" in "K A L"). The few patients who have had attentional dyslexia have had large tumors that occupied posterior regions of the left hemisphere and extended into subcortical structures. The rarity of the disorder makes the precise location of dam-age difficult to specify at present.

In contrast to visual word-form dyslexias, central dyslexias are thought to include reading processes that occur after the initial visual processing of words (McCarthy & Warrington, 1990). The two major types of central dyslexias include reading by sound (*surface dyslexia*, or phonological reading) and reading by sight vocabulary (with a corresponding inability to sound out words). Surface dylexia is a problem because of the abundance of words that defy the rules of regular letter–sound correspondences (e.g., "yacht," "busy," "sew," etc.). Because of their overreliance on pronunciation rules, surface dyslexics are likely to pronounce irregular words in predictable ways (e.g. "sew" as "sue") and also to pronounce phonologically regular pseudowords quite well (e.g., "blean"). Anatomically, surface dyslexia has been associated with a wide range of lesion locations, but usually tends to involve damage to the temporal lobes in conjunction with damage to other areas.

The second type of central dyslexia consists of being able to read using one's sight vocabulary but losing the ability to read by sound. In contrast to surface dyslexics, such patients are very poor at reading pseudowords that obey the spelling–sound rules of their language (e.g., "blean" or "tweal"). In addition, patients with the latter disorder may also have difficulty reading function words (e.g., "if," "for," etc.), grammatical morphemes (e.g., "-ed" or "-ing"), or abstract words (e.g., "idea"), and they sometimes make semantic errors as well. The co-ocurrence of pronunciation difficulty and difficulty with abstract words has been called *deep dyslexia*. Case studies of such patients reveal no consistent pattern of localization (Warrington & McCarthy, 1990). For example, several patients had large temporoparietal lesions and others had damage to the parieto-occipital region.

The late Norman Geschwind tried to summarize the literature on acquired dyslexias in the form of the anatomical model presented in Figure 6.2 (e.g., Geschwind & Galaburda, 1987). As can be seen, this model suggests that a written word is first registered in the primary visual areas of the occipital lobe. Activity in the visual area is then relayed to the angular gyrus, which is thought to play an important role in associating a visual form with a corresponding auditory representation in Wernicke's area. Activity then passes from Wernicke's area to Broca's area by way of a bundle of fibers called the *arcuate fasciculus*. If the person is reading aloud, signals are then sent from Broca's area to the primary motor cortex, which controls the movements of the lips, tongue, and so on.

What can be made of the aforementioned findings on the reading problems of brain-damaged adults? Two conclusions seem warranted. First, reading consists of multiple tasks that are performed in concert. For example, there are processes related to (1) perceiving letters and groups of letters; (2) pronunciation of word and letter strings; (3) syntactic processing related to function words and word endings; (4) semantic processes related to retrieving word meanings; and (5) conceptual processes related to the abstract–concrete continuum. Second, these pro-

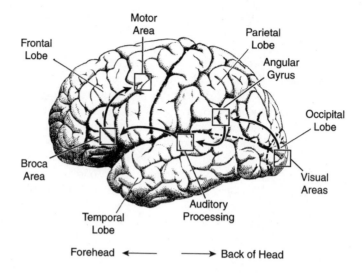

FIGURE 6.2. Brain areas corresponding to the Geschwind–Galaburda model.

cesses seem to be at least weakly modular and redundant (Kosslyn &
Koenig, 1992). That is, dyslexic individuals can read some words at least
some of the time despite their problems (e.g., surface dyslexics can read
phonologically regular words). Moreover, what they can do can overcompensate for what they cannot do (Stanovich & Siegel, 1994).

The findings from studies of dyslexic children (using standard laboratory tasks) and studies of normal adults using PET scans tend to corroborate and extend the findings from studies of brain-injured adults. In
particular, a large number of studies have revealed that the vast majority
of dyslexic children have the following characteristics: (1) they have a
great deal of difficulty pronouncing pseudowords; (2) they have difficulty on phonological tasks that do not require overt pronunciation; and
(3) they show relative strength in orthographic processing skill (Stanovich & Siegel, 1994). Hence, they are more like brain-injured adults
who have deep dyslexia than adults who have surface dyslexia.

Given the nature of children's problems, it is not surprising that
neuroscientists who study developmental dyslexia have tried to identify
morphological abnormalities in areas of the left temporal lobe that seem
to be responsible for phonological processing (Hynd, Marshall, & Gonzales, 1991). It should be noted, however, that classification systems that
are used for acquired dyslexias may not be appropriate for developmental dyslexias (Rayner & Pollatsek, 1989). With acquired dyslexias, there

are known sites of brain damage; the existence of damage in developmental dyslexia remains speculative (Reschly & Gresham, 1989). In addition, the practice of superimposing the categories of acquired dyslexia onto individuals with developmental dyslexia can hinder the discovery of the problems and mechanisms that are unique to developmental dyslexia (Raynor & Pollatsek, 1989). Further, it was noted earlier that deep dyslexia has not been associated with damage to particular sites in the brains of adults. If deep dyslexia in adults is, in fact, similar to developmental dyslexia in its manifest symptoms, it is not clear why developmentalists would expect to find abnormalities in particular sites in the brains of children.

Notwithstanding these caveats, Shaywitz and colleagues have recently used fMRI technology to determine whether different patterns of brain activity can be observed in the brains of dyslexic children and nondisabled children when they read (e.g., Shaywitz et al., 1998). Focusing on the regions identified by Geschwind (see Figure 6.2), they found that brain activations differed significantly between the two groups, with dyslexic readers showing relative underactivation in the striate cortex, angular gyrus, and Wernicke's area, and relative overactivation in the Broca area. Whereas these authors suggest that this pattern of activation might be a "signature" for dyslexia, it should be noted that involvement of left frontal areas is also indicative of task difficulty and working memory (Barch et al., 1997). To show that the aforementioned pattern really is a sign of functional disruption in the reading circuitry, these researchers would need to demonstrate at least two additional things in future studies: (1) that the pattern is not observed in nondyslexic children who are given a task that is hard for them and (2) that the pattern is not found in nondisabled children who are just beginning to read (who might have as much trouble pronouncing new words as older dyslexic children).

With respect to PET scan studies of normal adults, Posner et al. (1988) and Petersen, Fox, Snyder, and Raichle (1990) have found that passively looking at real words (e.g., "board"), pseudowords (e.g., "floop"), nonwords (e.g., "jvjfc"), and strings of letter-like fonts all activate the same portions of the occipital lobe. However, real words and pseudowords also activate portions of the occipital lobe that are not activated by nonwords and false fonts (the extrastriate cortex). Recall that damage to occipital regions often produces the visual word-form dyslexias that were described earlier. Whereas presentation of real words and being asked to define words activates regions of the left frontal lobe, presentation of pseudowords does not activate these regions. Finally, auditory and phonological processing seem to activate regions of the left temporal and lower parietal cortices, both of which are near regions of interest to individuals who study developmental dyslexia.

Collectively, then, a variety of neuroscientific studies have supported the idea that there are specific brain regions associated with orthographic, phonological, semantic, and syntactic processing. Orthographic processing seems to be centered in the primary visual area and the extrastriate area. Phonological processing seems to be associated with the superior temporal lobes and the angular gyrus (though Shaywitz and colleagues have also found frontal activation for rhyming tasks). Semantic processing has been associated with two regions in the left hemisphere: the Broca area (frontal lobe) and areas in the medial temporal lobe. The Broca area has also been associated with syntactic processing (Just & Carpenter, 1987). For example, patients diagnosed with Broca's aphasia have been found to have trouble with function words (e.g., "if," "for," etc.) and in recognizing the difference between sentence pairs such as the following:

- They gave her dog the biscuits.
- They gave her the dog biscuits.

Understanding the Causes and Neural Basis of Developmental Dyslexia

In Chapter 4, we learned that researchers who study attention-deficit/ hyperactivity disorder (ADHD) have been hampered by the fact that the definition of this disorder keeps changing (in part because ADHD is still poorly understood). Comparable definitional problems plague researchers who study reading disabilities. For example, most school systems assign the label "reading disabled" when there seems to be a discrepancy between a child's intelligence and his or her reading level (i.e., normal IQ but reading 2 years behind grade level). In recent years, this approach has been found to mix together two very different groups of children: those who have an actual reading disability and those who have been dubbed "garden variety" poor readers (Stanovich, 1988b). Whereas the latter can be brought up to speed through a short period of intense tutoring (e.g., 6 weeks), the former cannot (Vellutino et al., 1996). Further, comparisons of these two groups show marked differences in their phonological processing skills but no substantial differences in their visual, semantic, or syntactic skills (Vellutino et al., 1996; Stanovich & Siegel, 1994). The key problem here is that the discrepancy approach is not sensitive enough to pick up this phonological core deficit. In addition, use of this approach in longitudinal studies (e.g., Shaywitz, Escobar, Shaywitz, Fletcher, & Makuch, 1992), reveals four kinds of children: (1) those who meet the discrepancy criterion at both of two testings (2%), (2) those who meet the criterion at the first testing but not at the second testing (6%), (3) those who are said to be nondisabled at the first testing but reading disabled at the second testing (7%), and (4) those found to be nondisabled at both testings (85%). If the discrepancy approach were sufficiently accurate, the second group should not appear. After all, a child who catches up after a few years of instruction is probably not really disabled.

In the literature, some researchers have taken pains to make sure that their sample only includes children with authentic reading disabilities. Most others, however, have relied on the discrepancy criteria employed by children's school systems. This difference in definitions makes comparisons across studies difficult. To believe some set of findings (e.g., that dyslexic children demonstrate less blood flow to a certain region of the brain than good readers), we have to believe that the labels applied to children in a given study (i.e., "dyslexic" vs. "normal reader") are accurate.

A second issue relates to the anatomy of reading disability. Let's consider for a moment some of the ways in which the brains of reading-disabled and nondisabled children could differ. From the neuroscientific literature, it has been suggested that the following brain areas (at least) are involved in reading written material: the primary visual area, the extrastriate cortex, the left angular gyrus, the medial and superior regions of the left temporal lobe, Broca's area and surrounding left frontal areas, and the primary motor area. Based on arguments presented in Chapter 2, it can be said that these areas will only function properly if they contain a sufficient number of the right kind of neurons that are configured in the right way. In addition, for the whole system to work properly, each area needs to be appropriately connected to one or more of the other areas though long fibers (e.g., the *arcuate fasciculus*).

The quest for anatomical differences between disabled and nondisabled readers requires that we can tell when someone has the right number and right type of neurons connected in the right way. But to imagine the difficulty of this task, consider the following analogy. In order for a regiment in an army to carry out some mission, there has to be the right number and type of specialists (e.g., soldiers who can do reconnaissance, soldiers who can fire large artillery, etc.). Few people could look at a regiment marching by and say whether it had the right number and type of specialists. In the same way, it would be rather difficult for most scientists to look at microscopic slices of brain tissue and know whether the right number of neural elements were in place. Sometimes too few neurons could be the problem. Other times, however, too many neurons could be the problem.

In addition, if the neuroanatomy of reading really is a system of interdependent parts, problems could conceivably arise if something were wrong with any (or several) of the brain regions described above (in the same way that a tight-knit, interdependent baseball team might start to lose if any of its starters were to be injured). Thus, the search for the key area of disruption may be misguided. In addition, the idea that there seems to be built-in redundancy in the reading system suggests that more than one area would have to be affected in order for an intractable reading problem to emerge.

With all of these issues of definition and anatomy in mind, we can now examine several recent proposals regarding the etiology of reading disabilities from a more informed perspective. The first proposal arose in response to three sets of findings: (1) a higher incidence of language problems in boys, (2) symmetry or reversed asymmetry in the size of certain brain areas in dyslexic children, and (3) unexpected empirical links between left-handedness, language disorders, and immune disorders (Geschwind & Behan, 1982; Geschwind & Galaburda, 1985). To explain all of these findings, Geschwind and colleagues proposed the following. During prenatal development, testosterone levels affect the growth of the left cerebral hemisphere in such a way that an anomalous form of dominance develops. Instead of being right-handed and having language lateralized in the left hemisphere (the most common kind of dominance pattern), affected individuals become left-handed with language lateralized in the right or in both hemispheres. This altered physiology, in turn, leads to problems such as developmental dyslexia, impaired language development, and autism. Testosterone levels also affect the thymus, resulting in disorders of the immune system (e.g., allergies, colitis, AIDS).

In early formulations, the elevated level of testosterone was thought to retard the development of the left hemisphere such that it fails to show the typical pattern (in 66% of people) of growing larger than the right hemisphere. In later proposals (e.g., Galaburda, 1993), however, the suggestion of retarded growth of the left hemisphere was replaced with the idea that something interferes with normal *reductions* in the size of the right hemisphere (e.g., testosterone inhibits the process of cell death). Either way, both proposals were meant to explain the finding mentioned above that 66% of dyslexic children tend to have either symmetric brains or reversed asymmetry (right larger than left). The region of particular interest in these studies was the *planum temporale* (located bilaterally at the posterior portion of the superior surface of the temporal lobe). The location of the plana suggested that this region may have something to do with phonological processing, a particular problem for children with dyslexia and language delay.

Although the Geschwind–Behan–Galaburda (GBG) proposal showed some early promise, comprehensive meta-analyses have recently revealed numerous anomalies in the literature (Beaton, 1997; Bryden, McManus, & Bulman-Fleming, 1994). The first problem is that the incidence of reading problems may not really be higher in boys than girls. Boys are simply more likely to be referred for services than girls, reflecting a bias of teachers and other school personnel (Shaywitz, Shaywitz, Fletcher, & Escobar, 1990). Second, studies that have tried to show the three-way relation between left-handedness, immune disorders, and dyslexia have failed to find this relation. Third, the asymmetry of the plana may have more to do with handedness than with language lateralization. Fourth, the human species may rely less on cell death than other species to sculp brains (see Chapter 2). Finally, there is no hard evidence that sex hormones affect human brain structure (see Chapter 2). Problems such as these led Bryden et al. (1994, p. 155) to conclude their review of the literature on the GBG model by saying: "All things considered, we find the evidence to support the [GBG] model lacking and would suggest that psychologists and physicians have more useful things to do than carry out further assessments of the model."

But if the GBG model is incorrect, what else could explain the hard-to-remediate problems of dyslexic children? In other words, if symmetry or reversed symmetry in the plana is not the problem, what is wrong with dyslexic children's reading circuitry and how did it get that way? Several groups of researchers have begun to explore the possibility that reading problems are genetically determined. Studies suggest that 23–65% of children who have a parent with dyslexia also have the disorder. The rate among siblings can run as high as 40% (Shaywitz, 1996). In a longitudinal study of twins, DeFries et al. (1993) found that 53.5% of MZ twins were concordant for reading problems, compared to just 31.5% of DZ twins. Subsequent linkage studies have implicated loci on chromosomes 6 and 15 (Gayan et al., 1999).

Although these findings are intriguing, it is important to note that all of the aforementioned studies relied on such things as school records and self-reports to indicate the presence of reading problems within families. It is not clear how many of the children and adults in these studies were truly dyslexic and how many were simply "garden variety" poor readers. Second, estimates of the heritability of reading problems suggest that nongenetic (i.e., environmental) factors account for more than half (56%) of the variance (DeFries et al., 1993). Third, reading problems may not be encoded in a person's genes per se. Instead, there may be a genetic susceptibility to problems in translating genetic instructions into a specific anatomy (e.g., problems in proliferation, migration, or synaptogenesis processes; see Chapter 2). Finally, the fact that reading has a genetic component tells us nothing about the nature of the neurological underpinnings of dyslexia. In other words, we still do not know what is wrong with a dyslexic individual's neural circuitry and how it got that way. Moreover, the fact that the concordance rate for reading problems in identical twins is less than 100% implies that epigenetic and environmental factors must be also involved.

To better understand the role of genetics in reading problems, it may be helpful to consider the following analogy. The problems encountered in building a brain from genetic instructions may be similar to the problems encountered when someone builds a house from a blueprint. Consider how easy it would be for an incompetent contractor to construct a poorly built house from a perfectly fine blueprint. Conversely, note how a good contractor can sometimes build a sound house even when he or she is given a flawed set of blueprints. If reading problems really are encoded in a person's genes, perhaps there are ways to build a nondisabled brain from this flawed set of genetic instructions. The latter must be true given the concordance data from MZ twins described above. If both twins have flawed instructions, why is it that only one twin ends up having reading problems? And given the probabilistic nature of the gene–brain connection, would it not be possible for a reading-disabled brain to arise from a "perfectly fine" set of genetic blueprints?

Is There a Neuroscientific Basis to Reading Readiness and Precocious Reading?

The following discussion of reading readiness and precocious reading builds on the prior discussion of reading disability. Throughout the recent history of reading instruction (dating back to the turn of the century), there has been the pervasive suggestion that reading has a maturational component to it. In particular, many educators have assumed that it is not possible to teach reading to children until they are maturationally "ready" to benefit from this instruction. Some went so far as to use IQ tests to determine when the brain was ready (Morphett & Washburn, 1931). In the 1960s, the idea of maturational readiness was further fueled by intense interest in the stage theory of Jean Piaget. Many educators misread Piaget's theory to suggest that (1) knowledge growth was biologically based and (2) children could not be taught to read until they were in Piaget's third stage of intellectual development ("concrete operations"). In point of fact, Piaget explicitly argued against maturational accounts (e.g., Gesell, Chomsky, etc.) and appealed to knowledge-based constraints on intellectual development instead (Byrnes, 2001). Moreover, he had nothing to say about reading, despite the fact that he wrote hundreds of works over the span of 60 years.

Nevertheless, it is common for teachers and parents to report that their preschoolers vigorously resist being taught to read. In addition, experimental and informal attempts to teach children how to read have generally failed when children are below the age of 5 (Feitelson, Tehori, & Levinberg-Green, 1982; Fowler, 1971). There are, however, documented cases of precocious readers who ranged in age from 2 to 5 when they began reading (Fowler, 1971; Goldstein, 1978; Jackson, 1992), as well as a few experimental programs that have been seemingly successful with 4- and 5-year-olds (Feitelson et al., 1982; Fowler, 1971). If we combine this evidence with the fact that it is often straightforward to teach (nondisabled) working-class and middle-class 6-year-olds to read, it seems perfectly reasonable to suspect that something neurological might be going on.

However, well-controlled studies have found that age alone is not a very good predictor of responsiveness to reading instruction when factors related to knowledge and experience are taken into account (Adams, 1990; Bryant, MacLean, Bradley, & Crossland, 1990; Stanovich & Siegel, 1994). Early studies (e.g., Fowler, 1971; Morphett & Washburn, 1931) showed that it was a child's *mental age*, not his or her chronological age, that mattered (e.g., a 2-year-old who could answer 5-year-old questions on an IQ test could learn to read better than a 5-year-old who could only answer 4-year-old questions). Mental age and intelligence were soon replaced in later studies with two better predictors: the speed with which children could name letters (letter knowledge) and the ability to reflect on and manipulate speech sounds (phonemic awareness). Children are clearly not born with knowledge of letters and they need to acquire a substantial receptive vocabulary (through experience) in order to create segmented, phonetic representations of spoken words (Metsala, 1999). Segmented representations, in turn, are required for creating links between graphemes and phonemes. Thus, a lack of receptivity to instruction could reflect a lack of exposure to relevant information. Similarly, it is no coincidence that precocious readers usually come from affluent, well-educated homes and that 4-year-olds who learn to read have unusually high levels of letter knowledge for 4-year-olds (e.g., Fowler, 1971). Moreover, middle-class children have an easier time learning to read in the first grade than disadvantaged children (of all races) because the latter enter school with lower levels of letter knowledge and phonemic awareness (Byrnes, 2001).

Thus, it would appear that age constraints on reading instruction reflect the fact that it takes time for children to acquire important kinds of knowledge (i.e., knowledge of letter names and segmented phonetic representations of words). This knowledge, of course, must be embodied in the form of neural assemblies (i.e., clusters of neural groups that have formed synaptic connections with each other). In order for neural assemblies to form, there has to be a sufficient number of neurons located in certain regions of the brain that have matured to the point that they can form synaptic connections with neighbors. Studies of brain development suggest that only the neurons in the frontal lobe continue to develop substantially beyond infancy, so the primary temporal constraint related to maturation may well be the time it takes for synapses to form after repeated encounters with the same kind of stimulation (e.g., the sight of a given letter). But if Shaywitz and colleagues are right that frontal areas are somehow disabled in poor readers (and important for phonemic awareness), then perhaps there may be two kinds of factors that explain why it is hard to teach children below the age of 4 to read: (1) experiential factors (e.g., insufficient exposure to letters and spoken words) and (2) maturational factors (e.g., continued development of frontal brain regions).

CONCLUSIONS, CAVEATS, AND INSTRUCTIONAL IMPLICATIONS

As a means of summarizing and drawing implications from the preceding discussion of reading, I shall consider answers to the following four questions:

1. How much overlap is there between the psychological and neuroscientific accounts of reading?
2. Is it possible to fuse these accounts into a single integrated perspective?
3. How confident can we be in the portrait of reading that has emerged from these two traditions?
4. When and how should children be taught to read, given what we have learned from these two traditions?

The Overlap Question

As I have noted several times in this book, psychologists conduct studies to find support for particular theoretical models (which "carve" psychological entities into their components). An excellent example of such a carving would be the model of skilled reading shown in Figure 6.1. The neuroscientific approach, in contrast, is often more concerned with revealing clusters of behavioral symptoms than with testing a particular theoretical model (i.e., the patient does X when asked to point to a word and Y when asked to read it aloud). This basic difference in orientation means that sometimes there can be very little overlap between accounts that emerge from the psychological versus the neuroscientific perspectives.

In practice, however, accounts from these two perspectives often do overlap for three reasons (see Chapters 3 and 4). First, neuroscientists are not just interested in case studies. They are also interested in associating brain regions with the components of some cognitive skill. As such, they often use psychological theories to get a sense of what these components might be. Second, psychologists are not just interested in normal behavior. They are also interested in the extremes (exceptionally high and low performers) and in individual differences. Scholars who focus on such issues inevitably seem to entertain brain-based explanations of these differences. Third, many psychologists have recently come to appreciate the fact that neuroscientific evidence can be used to support a favored theoretical carving.

It is for all three reasons that the psychological and neuroscientific literatures on reading seem to overlap a great deal. There is, for example, converging evidence from both camps in support of the claim that reading involves orthographic, semantic, syntactic, and phonological processing. Similarly, Seidenberg and McClelland's psychological model (Figure 6.1) is very compatible with Geschwind's anatomical model (Figure 6.2). Inasmuch as the former model was intentionally based on the notion of "brain-style" computation, this compatibility makes a great deal of sense.

Nonetheless, a number of psychological notions have yet to find counterparts in the neuroscience of reading. For example, how are schemata represented in the brain? Are such representations localized to particular regions of the brain or are they widely distributed? Similarly, which brain structures are active when a child is engaged in letter-naming and phonemic analysis tasks? Why might these regions be related to reading readiness? In addition, to what extent are imagery processes in the right parietal lobes involved in the construction of situation models? Where are reading strategies (e.g., inference making and backtracking) carried out in the brain?

The Integration Question

It is only a matter of time before we will know whether scholars can provide consistent and credible answers to the questions posed in the preceding section. If such answers do emerge, we will be in a better position to know whether the psychological perspective on reading can be fused with the neuroscientific perspective. The integration can be said to have progressed substantially when (1) the two perspectives converge on the same componential analysis (e.g., both settle on something like the Seidenberg and McClelland model) and (2) the neuroscientific bases of reading development and reading disabilities are well understood.

The Confidence Question

As implied in the previous section, psychologists and neuroscientists seem to be converging on highly similar portraits of reading. How confident can we be that this consensus portrait is accurate? One way to address this question is to consider the kinds of proposals that could be overturned by new data and the kinds that could not, or probably will not, be. For example, there is little reason to think that new evidence will make the idea of orthographic processing obsolete. People have to be able to recognize the written symbols of their language. However, it is possible that a particular *model* of orthographic processing (i.e., the connectionist idea of units) could be found to be inaccurate. In addition, it is also possible that scientists have not discovered all of the component operations of reading. In other words, another oval or two may have to be added to the model shown in Figure 6.1. The fact that animals cannot be used in experimental studies also causes problems because we may never get to the level of neuronal specificity enjoyed by scientists who have studied development, memory, or attention. Finally, some of the conclusions drawn by neuroscientists have been clouded by the fact that researchers have not always used the most sensitive measures of reading disability. In addition, many neuroimaging studies rely on the processing of single words. It is not clear what brain regions would be active if people were to read lengthier, realistic segments of connected text.

Thus, despite the fact that reading has been the subject of investigation since the late 19th century, there is still the chance that certain fundamental assumptions could change as new evidence comes in from psychological and neuroscientific studies. It may be best, then, to remain only moderately confident in the portrait of reading that has emerged so far.

Instructional Implications

Let's assume for the moment that (1) reading does, in fact, involve schemata, strategies, and the processors shown in Figure 6.1, and that (2) neuroscientists have identified most of the brain regions associated with reading. How should reading be taught to children, given what psychologists and neuroscientists have discovered at this point? When should reading instruction begin?

The first point to make is that there is a fundamental gap between any given theoretical carving and instructional practice. Teachers, for example, need to know more than the fact that reading involves four processors in order to know how to promote reading skills in their students. They also need to know how to *promote the development of these four processors and their interconnections.* The Seidenberg and McClelland model is based on the idea of associations that develop through repetition and practice. Does this mean that teachers should engage in meaningless rote learning using flashcards? Not necessarily. Practice and repetition must surely be involved, but it need not be meaningless and boring. Kids who play video games learn a lot about the components of, and characters in, these games through repetition, but they do not mind or even notice the repetition. Also, recall the finding that pseudowords given a meaning are processed faster than meaningless pseudowords. One thing that we have seemed to learn about reading, then, is that it involves multiple, redundant components that should be promoted in tandem. There is little support for the idea of separating out a component skill and working on that skill in isolation. Thus, contemporary psychological and neuroscientific research suggests that it would be ill-advised to either exclusively focus on phonics and spelling instruction (to the neglect of meaning), or exclusively focus on whole words and meaning (to the exclusion of spelling and phonics). In other words, approaches that combine the best of whole language and phonics approaches find support in both the psychological and the neuroscientific literatures on reading.

A related point pertains to the construct of reading disability. If we were to find out that reading-disabled children have, say, inadequate reciprocal connections between the left frontal and temporal lobes, what implications would this have for the best way to teach reading-disabled children? Whereas some teachers would give up on reading-disabled children after learning this information (i.e., they would assume that there is no hope for these children because there is something wrong with their brains), others might reason that they should teach to the brain areas that still "work" well (e.g. visual areas) in the hopes that strong visual skills might compensate for weaker phonological processing. Still others might reason that reading-disabled children simply need more practice in order to eventually get up to a functional level. In other words, their neurological problems makes their learning painfully slow, but they will eventually get to where they need to be. Note how all three responses are to the same piece of information. Note also that teachers could differ further even if they responded in the same way to information that there was something specifically wrong with the brains of reading-disabled children. For example, one teacher who responds in the third way above (that children will eventually get up to speed) might engage in endless hours of flashcards while the other uses a more interesting approach (e.g., computerized reading games).

The final points pertain to the issue of when reading instruction should begin. Children do not have much of a vocabulary before age 2 (including names for letters). Moreover, they have to be capable of understanding and hearing individual sounds as well as to understand the fact that writers associate sounds with letters. Such forms of knowledge take time to acquire, and there may be neurological developments in the frontal lobes to consider (as noted earlier). Thus, there is good reason to suspect that reading instruction would be relatively ineffective before the age of 3 or 4. But even if it could be shown that the cognitive brain is ready to learn reading by age 3, for example, there is also that matter of children's interest and motivation. Just because we *can* teach something to very young children does not mean that we *should* teach it to them. But it would be extremely unwise not to teach reading skills in some form to older 4- and 5-year-olds. One of the best ways to promote academic success in a child is to have him or her begin first grade as a fairly competent reader. Again, though, the question of when is different than the question of how. There are interesting and playful ways to promote reading skills and boring, formal ways.

CHAPTER 7

Math Skills

Throughout the school year, children are asked to take a variety of aptitude tests, achievement tests, and teacher-made tests. For the most part, teachers and administrators use these tests in order to gauge their students' learning, place students into various ability groups, or determine the effectiveness of particular instructional techniques. For hundreds of years, it has been observed that test scores often array themselves into a characteristic bell-shaped distribution; that is, about one-sixth of students score below average, two-thirds score near the average, and one-sixth score above the average (Bernstein, 1996). This low-to-high performance continuum is thought to occur because (1) most tests are intentionally designed to identify the "actual" level of talent or mastery in each student and (2) students tend to differ in the amount of ability they seem to possess, or the amount of content they seem to master in a given time period (due to differences in effort, differing levels of access to adequate instruction, differing levels of talent, or various combinations of these factors). If all students received the same scores each time a test was given, the issue of ability would probably fall into the background of everyday existence and scientific enterprises. In other words, we all would probably not even think about abilities. The fact that scores always seem to vary, however, pushes the constructs of ability (and individual differences in these abilities) to the forefront of most people's consciousness. In recent years, it has been claimed that children and adults notice these differences (and other variations in the environment) because the human mind is "built" to see them and naturally motivated to want to explain them (Pinker, 1997). Whereas scientists construct formal theories to explain variations in ability and other kinds of variations, nonscientists are thought to create so-called naive or folk theories.

145

In this chapter, I shall examine several scientific theories regarding the nature of mathematical abilities. In the first section, my focus is on psychological accounts that were constructed to explain the variations in performance that occur on classroom tests, standardized tests, or experimenter-made tests. This psychological view is supplemented by a related view that has recently emerged from the field of mathematics education. Scholars in the latter field have often gained their inspiration from psychological accounts, but they also have elaborated on these accounts using classroom experiences, expert models, and logical argumentation as guides. In the second section, my focus is on neuroscientific accounts that were constructed to explain the variations in performance that occur when the following groups have been compared: (1) neurologically intact individuals versus individuals who have known brain injuries or mathematical disabilities, (2) students with high mathematical talent versus students with lower amounts of math talent, and (3) males versus females. In the final section, I assess the compatibility of the psychological and neuroscientific perspectives, and describe the instructional implications of an integrated account.

PSYCHOLOGICAL AND EDUCATIONAL PERSPECTIVES ON MATHEMATICAL ABILITIES

To a large extent, psychologists have tried to answer the following question: What is the nature of mathematical ability? Their answers to this question have tended to be theoretical (i.e., componential) descriptions of what it means to have math skills. In contrast, educators have usually sought answers to slightly different questions. For example, they have often asked, What *should* students know and be able to do in math when they graduate from high school? Thus, the math education perspective tends to be both *de*scriptive and *pre*scriptive.

When these two perspectives are synthesized, they suggest that mathematical ability involves the following components:

Declarative Knowledge

As I noted in Chapter 3, a person's declarative knowledge is his or her knowledge of the facts in some field. In the present case, declarative knowledge would refer to a person's knowledge of math facts (Byrnes, 2001). In most people, these facts amount to the answers to various computations (e.g., knowing that 9 is the right answer to 3×3, or that 25 is the square root of 625). Individuals who have considerable math talent usually know a number of math facts that are highly accessible (i.e., it does not take a long time for them to retrieve these facts). However, in recent years, this aspect of mathematical expertise has been downplayed in its importance (especially in the math education community) because people can have considerable knowledge of facts but still lack the ability to solve problems in the classroom or in the real world. In effect, declarative knowledge is thought to be a necessary but not sufficient condition for math talent (Byrnes, 1992).

Procedural Knowledge

A *procedure* is a set of operations or actions that is implemented to achieve some goal (Anderson, 1993; Byrnes, 2001). Thus, a person who has procedural knowledge in math knows how to achieve certain ends using a series of actions, operations, or steps. Examples include knowing how to (1) count an array of objects; (2) add, subtract, multiply, or divide whole numbers, fractions, integers, or algebraic symbols; (3) determine the area under a curve; (4) set up and carry out a geometric proof; and (5) use statistics to determine whether a correlation is significantly larger than zero. As I implied earlier, regular use of certain procedures on a finite set of mathematical objects (e.g., whole numbers between 1 and 20) yields answers that will ultimately comprise one portion of a person's declarative knowledge base. Moreover, certain forms of procedures have a "syntax" (Hiebert & LeFevre, 1987) in the sense that the steps must be performed in a certain way in order for correct answers to emerge (e.g., lining up the decimal points when manually adding numbers with decimals).

Psychologists and educators further assume that procedures can exist in the mind at different levels of abstraction (Byrnes, 1999). At the lowest level of abstraction, for example, are specific actions or algorithms (e.g., the actions involved in frying an egg or adding two fractions). These actions are "specific" in the sense that they apply to a limited range of objects and situations. For example, a person would presumably not attempt to crack open a hamburger before frying it or add negative integers with the least common denominator method.

At a somewhat higher level of abstraction are strategies and heuristics. A *strategy* is a plan that (1) describes, in outline, how a problem will be approached and (2) includes some specification of the overall goal (e.g., find out what angle X is) and the subgoals that need to be achieved in order to attain the overall goal (e.g., First I need to find out. . . . Then I have to. . . .). Strategies are more abstract than action-based procedures because the former may be formulated well before particular methods for attaining each subgoal are even envisioned. Moreover, the same general strategy may be applied in a variety of situations. A related kind of procedural knowledge is a *heuristic*, or a rule of thumb (e.g., "When in doubt, ask the teacher").

An interesting aspect of the research on math strategies is the finding that children and adults seem to rely on a repertoire of five to seven strategies to solve even structurally similar problems (Siegler, 1991b). For example, for the problem "3 + 7," a child may count out three using one hand, count out seven using the other hand, then add up all the extended fingers (the *count-all* strategy). For the problem "18 + 2," however, the same child may start counting at the largest number, then add two numbers onto that (the *min* strategy). The general approach is to use strategies that are not only efficient but likely to yield the correct answer.

In sum, then, psychologists and educators assume that mathematical ability requires a rich procedural knowledge base. However, again it is not enough to simply have facts, procedures, strategies, and heuristics stored in long-term memory. Mathematical competence involves the ability to call on the *right* facts, procedures, and strategies at the *right* time. The component to be described next has been alleged to support this kind of context-sensitive use.

Conceptual Knowledge

As I implied in Chapter 3, people would be expected to develop conceptual knowledge in math as they (1) struggle to understand the *meaning* of mathematical facts and procedures, (2) learn to relate mathematical symbols to their referents and construct categories of mathematical entities, and (3) construct cardinal and ordinal representations of mathematical entities (Byrnes, 2001; Case & Okamoto, 1996). Clearly, there is a critical difference between knowing certain facts and knowing *why* these facts are true. Similarly, there is a difference between knowing how to execute a procedure and knowing why it should be performed in a particular instance (and why it should be executed in a particular way). Individuals with conceptual knowledge understand the meaning and appropriate use of mathematical facts and procedures. Moreover, they relate various mathematical symbols to their referents in appropriate ways (in the same way that literate individuals relate words to their referents). The latter skill requires the construction of mathematical categories and definitions (e.g., *odd number, integer, rational number, integral*, etc.). One particularly important type of categorical representation for math is called a *schema* (plural, *schemata*).

Schemata are abstract representations of what all instances of something (e.g., word problems that require addition) have in common. Schemata form through repeated encounters with the same kind of problem or situation, especially when analogous or identical solutions are required (Byrnes, 2001; Mayer, 1982). When problems are recognized as being of a particular type, their solutions can be immediately retrieved instead of having to be reinvented on the spot. Hence, schemata probably provide the basis of *conditional knowledge*, knowing when and where to apply a procedure. However, certain theoretical models of procedural knowledge build conditions of use into the procedure itself.

The final kind of conceptual knowledge refers to the fused, linear representation of the cardinal and ordinal representations of mathematical quantities. Cardinal representations describe the amount or extent of a set of objects (i.e., how many objects might be present in a particular situation). When the cardinal representations for various quantities are arranged in increasing magnitude, a student can be said to have an ordinal representation of these numbers as well. An example would be a mental number line of integer amounts. To assess cardinal and ordinal knowledge, a researcher could present two arrays of objects and ask a person to identify the larger amount.

Thus, conceptual knowledge involves mappings of mental representations to things in the external world (so-called *extension relations*), as well as mappings between multiple representations in the mind (so-called *intension relations*). Together, these representations help a student understand and make sense of math facts and procedures. By "make sense," it is meant that a child truly understands "the big picture" when it comes to concepts as well as the likely effects of some procedures. For example, a student with math sense would appreciate what might happen if the 3 in $3 \times 4 = 12$ were to be replaced by a 4 and how such a change would be different from substituting a 4 for the 3 in $3 + 4 = 7$ (Byrnes, 2001; Markovits & Sowder, 1994). Hence, the child essentially knows what is going on in math class.

Moreover, the construction of mathematical categories helps a child to avoid inappropriate applications of procedures. For example, a child with conceptual knowledge of fractions would not simply add the numerators and denominators of two fractions together because the two categories of fractions and whole numbers are representationally distinct in their minds (Byrnes, 1992). Each of these categories, in turn, is linked to its own set of procedures. Whereas individuals with high math ability have large amounts of declarative, procedural, and conceptual knowledge of math, their less competent peers often only have declarative and procedural knowledge (if that). In other words, the latter may often do the right things but have no idea what they are doing or why.

Estimation Skills

Sometimes a problem requires only an approximate solution. For example, an employer may only wish to know the probable month (or even time of year) when a job will be completed, not the exact date. Or a homeowner may wish to get only a rough idea of how much a monthly payment would go down with refinancing, or how much money to bring to the supermarket. In such cases, a skilled individual needs to know how to use math facts, procedures, concepts, and strategies to generate an approximate but still useful solution. For example, consider the case of a third grader who wanted to know the approximate answer to the problem, $25 \times 25 = ?$. She may already know that 20×20 is 400 and that 30×30 is 900. From these two math facts and her ordinal representations of whole numbers (i.e., 25 is midway between 20 and 30), she may deduce that 25×25 is probably somewhere in between 400 and 900, and perhaps close to the halfway mark of 650 (again using ordinal representations or quick computations to determine the halfway mark). The estimate of 650 is, of course, reasonably close to the correct answer of 625. On important tests like the National Assessment of Educational Progress (NAEP) or the Scholastic Achievement Test (SAT), estimation skills are required for scoring in the highest ranges because most problems have to be solved in 60 seconds or less. Whereas approximate answers can be generated in a few seconds and be compared to possible answers, complete computations often take more than the allotted 60 seconds. Given earlier arguments, one could say that estimation skills are simply a form of math sense. It should also be clear that one could not be proficient at estimating without having large amounts of declarative, procedural, and conceptual knowledge in math. But again, there are students who have the latter kinds of knowledge but lack the ability or tendency to engage in estimation when it is appropriate to do so.

Graphing and Modeling Skills

Mathematics has often been said to be a discipline that can be used to identify patterns and functional relationships in the world. When data points are presented in a serial fashion or one by one, it is often difficult to get an overall sense of what is going on. For example, if a person wanted to get a rough sense of the housing prices in a given neighborhood, he or she could read an unorganized list of prices for the last 100 houses that sold in that neighborhood (one by one), but such an activity would not be very helpful. A better approach would be to make a bar graph or tally sheet to see where most of the prices fall (using prices arranged in increasing order along the bottom of the graph). Similarly, researchers in multiple fields use an approach called *regression* to see which of a set of predictor variables is statistically related to some outcome for a large sample of cases. For example, a scientist can use regression to predict someone's yearly income using variables such as age, occupation, and mortgage payment. Here, statistical programs in computers link up such variables in a mathematical function. This function indicates which variables are useful for prediction and which are not. The equations generated by the computer also indicate which variables (e.g., mortgage payments) are better predictors than others (e.g., age). Graphs, charts, and mathematical equations, then, help a person develop a good conceptual understanding of patterns in the data. These aides also reduce the amount of information processing that has to be performed to see the patterns and also greatly facilitate inference making (Bruner, 1966). People with high levels of math ability use graphic aides in a strategic fashion. Moreover, they rely on their extensive knowledge to create these models. Note that these tendencies reflect something other than spatial ability.

Problem Solving

To sum up, then, mathematical ability requires (1) high levels of declarative, procedural, and conceptual knowledge *and* (2) a tendency to use this knowledge in a strategic, efficient, and context-sensitive way. This analysis suggests that in a national sample of students, there would probably be four kinds of individuals. The first would be students who do not use math knowledge in a strategic, efficient, or context-sensitive way because they have low levels of declarative, procedural, and conceptual knowledge. The second would be students who have adequate levels of declarative and procedural knowledge but are unable to use this knowledge to solve problems due to the fact that they have insufficient levels of conceptual knowledge, were given inadequate guidance, or had too few opportunities to practice. The third would be students who have all three kinds of knowledge but do not use this knowledge to solve problems because of inadequate instruction or insufficient opportunities to practice. The final would be students who can solve a wide range of problems because they have the requisite knowledge, and have received multiple, guided opportunities to apply this knowledge.

NEUROSCIENTIFIC PERSPECTIVES ON MATH ABILITY

By and large, neuroscientists have attempted to explain mathematical abilities and disabilities by appealing to individual differences in the operation of specific brain mechanisms. In what follows, the neuroscientific literature on math skills is summarized in five sections. In the first, the focus is on several models of math skills that were constructed to explain the calculation deficits that sometimes occur following brain injury. In the second, the literature on math disabilities in children is summarized. In the third, neuroimaging studies of math skills are reviewed. In the fourth, the focus shifts from math disabilities to mathematical talent. In the fifth and final section, a summary of the neuroscientific literature is provided.

Neuroscientific Models of Calculation

Two models have recently been proposed to account for the patterns of calculation deficits that have sometimes occurred following brain injuries. For expository purposes, these theoretical frameworks are called the *McCloskey model* and the *Dehaene model*, respectively, though the focal individuals have had several collaborators.

The McCloskey Model

After conducting a detailed analysis of 14 case studies of brain-injured adults, Michael McCloskey and colleagues (e.g., McCloskey, Caramazza, & Basili, 1985; McCloskey, Aliminosa, & Sokol, 1991) proposed that calculation abilities can be decomposed into two clusters of functionally autonomous components. The first cluster, which comprise a *number processing system*, includes one set of components for comprehending numbers and another set for producing them. Within each of the comprehension and production subsystems, moreover, there are distinct components for processing arabic numbers (e.g., *53*) and verbal numbers (e.g., *fifty-three*). All of these components were originally proposed to account for various forms of double dissociations that appeared in the focal cases. For example, some of the patients could recognize arabic numbers but could not write them down when asked. Similarly, some could write down arabic numbers but not verbal numbers.

The components in the second cluster comprise the *calculation system*. McCloskey et al. (1985, 1991) argue that these components perform three kinds of processes: (1) comprehension of the signs or words for operations (e.g., ÷, *divided by*), (2) retrieval of arithmetic facts (e.g., that 39 is the answer to 13 × 3), and (3) execution of calculation procedures (e.g., the algorithm for long division). Again, these components were inferred on the basis of certain double dissociations. Some patients, for example, could recognize the signs for operations but could not perform the operations indicated by these signs. Others, however, could perform the operations, but could not retrieve math facts associated with these operations. Moreover, there were individuals who could do some of the operations from the calculation system but could not do others from the number processing system (McCloskey et al., 1991). When the two systems are intact, however, they are thought to be linked via the ability to create abstract representations of the numbers and operations in a problem. This abstract representation is also linked to action systems that are alleged to regulate the implementation of goal-directed procedures.

Beyond such double dissociations, five other interesting aspects of the 14 cases emerged. The first is that, in most of the patients (64%), problems developed after these patients experienced a cerebrovascular accident in the left hemisphere. In two other patients (14%), the cerebrovascular accident occurred in the right hemisphere. The remaining patients experienced a closed head injury (14%) or anoxia (7%). Thus, calculation skills in arithmetic seem to be localized in the left hemisphere, but the data are not completely consistent in this regard. These findings are, however, analogous to those that have been observed in postmortem studies of dyslexic children. In these studies, 66% of the children showed either symmetry or reversed asymmetry of the plana temporale (see Chapter 6). The rest showed the normal pattern of asymmetry. It is curious that in both cases, two-thirds of subjects showed problems in the same region of the brain, but one-third did not.

The second interesting finding was that in all 14 cases the calculation deficits were limited to multiplication (i.e., arithmetic skills for addition and subtraction were left largely intact). Thus, these findings suggest that there are brain regions associated with multiplication, and other regions associated with arithmetic and subtraction. The third finding was that all patients showed uneven patterns of performance across particular kinds of multiplication problems. For example, some patients could solve all problems except those involving zero (e.g., 3 × 0 or 0 × 4). Others could solve problems with zero when it was the first but not the second multiplicand. Still others had no problem with items involving zeros and ones (e.g., 3 x 0 and 1 x 4), but had problems with all other combinations that had multiplicands between 2 and 9. The fourth finding was that each person seemed to have problems with their own types of items. Such findings combined with related evidence from other case studies (e.g., Hittmair-Delazer, Semenza, & Denes, 1994) suggest that each fact seems to be stored in its own format. Further analysis showed that many patients forgot the facts associated with all types of problems but could quickly reconstruct the facts for the problems with zero or one because the more abstract rules for these items were spared (e.g., "any number multiplied by 1 is itself"). Thus, there seem to be brain regions that store such abstract rules and others that store other kinds of multiplication algorithms (e.g., how to line things up in columns for problems such as 317×32). This finding regarding the abstract rules has been replicated in other case studies (e.g., Pesenti, Seron, & Van Der Linden, 1994).

The Dehaene Model

Dehaene and Cohen (1997) reviewed the neuropsychological literature related to mathematical deficits and proposed a "triple-code" model to account for the myriad of findings. As the name implies, the triple-code model suggests that there are three main representations of numbers: (1) a *visual arabic code* that is localized in the left and right inferior occipital-temporal areas, (2) an *analogical quantity* or *magnitude code* that is localized in the left and right inferior parietal areas, and (3) a *verbal code* that is localized in the left perisylvian areas. The visual arabic code, which subserves multidigit operations, is utilized during the identification of strings of digits and during judgments of parity (e.g., knowing that numbers that end in 2 are even). The magnitude code, in contrast, is assumed to correspond to distributions of activation on an oriented number line. This code subserves the ability to evaluate proximity (e.g., that 18 is close to 20) and ordinal relations (e.g., that 20 is larger than 18). The verbal code, finally, represents numbers via a parsed sequence of words. It is involved when an individual accesses rote verbal memories of arithmetic facts.

Dehaene and Cohen further suggest that there are two basic routes through which arithmetic problems can be solved. In the direct route, the problem (e.g., 2×9) is first encoded into a verbal representation (e.g., "two times nine is . . . "). The verbal representation, in turn, triggers the rote-learned verbal answer that is stored in memory (e.g., "eighteen"). The latter process is thought to involve a left cortico–subcortical loop through the basal ganglia and thalamus. Hence, the direct route does not require conceptual analysis of any type and is largely devoid of meaning. In contrast, the second route is more indirect and calls on stored semantic knowledge of numbers. When problems are solved by the indirect route, a person recodes the arabic symbols into quantity representations. These quantity representations (thought to be localized in the left and right parietal areas) subserve semantically meaningful operations, such as when one alters a representation of the quantity 5 to make it into a representation of 7 or 3. The results of such manipulations are thought to be transmitted from the left inferior parietal cortex to the left perisylvian language network for naming.

Dehaene and Cohen's model, then, proposes that there are two major sets of brain areas that are critical for calculation: (1) the bilateral inferior parietal areas that are responsible for semantic knowledge about numerical quantities and (2) the left cortico–pallidum–thalamic loop that is involved in the storage of the verbal sequences that correspond to arithmetic facts. The model further assumes that brain lesions would have different effects depending on which of these two areas were damaged. The calculation deficits (or *acalculias*) that arise from damage to the inferior parietal areas should be domain-specific (i.e., damage should only affect number knowledge and not other kinds of knowledge) and be limited to problems that rely heavily on semantic math knowledge such as estimation, comparison, and ordinality (i.e., automatized facts should be uneffected). In contrast, acalculias that arise from damage to the cortico–subcortical loop should be domain-general (i.e., other kinds of rote-learned material besides math facts may be affected as well), and should involve loss of math facts combined with spared semantic skills (e.g., estimation, comparison, and ordinal relations).

Dehaene and Cohen (1997) demonstrated the utility of this model by applying it to two case studies. Whereas one of these patients had a localized inferior parietal lesion in the right hemisphere, the other had a left subcortical infarct. As predicted, the patient with the parietal lesion demonstrated the following double dissociation: he had difficulty considering semantic relations (e.g., comparing two numbers) but could recall automatized math facts. The other patient, in contrast, demonstrated the opposite kind of double dissociation.

Developmental Disabilities in Math

The aforementioned models were constructed to explain the calculation deficits that sometimes arise in brain-injured adults. Such acquired disabilities can be contrasted with so-called developmental disabilities in math (or MD). The latter term applies to problems that present themselves in children who have no known history of brain injury.

Children with MD have been found to have both procedural and fact-retrieval deficits. Moreover, these deficits appear to follow different developmental trajectories (Geary, 1993). In the case of procedural problems, for example, it has been found that children with MD usually lag behind their nondisabled peers in the sense that they often (1) use less mature strategies (e.g., "count all" vs. "min"), (2) perform the same strategies more slowly, and (3) make calculation errors more often. By the end of second grade, however, the computational skills of children with MD approach those of their non-MD peers. In contrast, fact-retrieval deficits tend to persist indefinitely and are resistant to remediation through extensive training. When children with MD attempt to recall facts, they tend to recall fewer facts, the retrieval times associated with these facts are very unsystematic, and they make a large number of retrieval errors (Geary, 1993).

It is notable that the two primary deficits of children with MD correspond to two of the three component operations of the calculation system proposed by McCloskey and colleagues (see above). The fact-retrieval problem is also consistent with aspects of Dehaene and Cohen's model. The research on which these models are based further suggests that procedural and fact-retrieval problems are particularly likely to arise following lesions to the left hemisphere or the left cortico–subcortical systems. This left hemisphere bias is interesting given the fact that 40% of the children who have MD have been found to have a reading disability as well (Geary, 1993). As we learned in Chapter 6, many important reading skills seem to be localized in the left hemisphere.

Studies Using Neuroimaging and Gross Electrical Recording Techniques

So far, the discussion has been limited to the math deficits that arise in disabled children and adults. In the present and next sections, the focus shifts somewhat to the math abilities of nonimpaired individuals. The two studies to be described next employed neuroimagining or gross electrical recording techniques while subjects performed math tasks. Studies of this sort are surprisingly rare (in contrast to the large number of neuroimagining studies of reading, attention, or memory).

Dehaene et al. (1996) presented number pairs to eight healthy adults. On one-third of the trials, subjects were asked to mentally identify the larger of the two numbers. On another third of trials, they were asked to multiply the two numbers together. On the remaining third of trials, they simply rested with their eyes open. Using PET scans, Dehaene et al. considered the differences in blood flow patterns that were evident when any of the two conditions were compared to each other (e.g., multiplying numbers vs. identifying the larger one). Results showed selective increases or decreases in blood flow in a number of brain areas. Notably, the number comparison task "did not yield any significant activations over and above those that . . . are related to stimulus identification and response selection (lateral occipital cortex, precentral gyrus, and [supplementary motor area]). . . . Hence, no critical brain areas for number comparison emerged" (Dehaene et al., 1996, p. 1103). Small activations, however, did emerge in the left and right inferior parietal region, but these activations were not significant (contrary to predictions based on Dehaene and Cohen's model; see above). It is not clear whether the use of PET scans, inadequate control trials, or a small sample size were responsible for these inconclusive results.

Using a 64-channel EEG technology (see Chapter 1), Dehaene (1996) limited his focus to just number identification and comparison. He attempted to verify a three-stage processing model that suggested that number comparison involved an initial stage of number comprehension (with distinct components for comprehending arabic and verbal symbols) that was followed by comparative processes that operate on the mental representations that emerge after the symbols are interpreted. Results suggested that arabic digits are initially comprehended bilaterally in posterior occipito–temporal regions. Verbal digits, however, seem to be processed mainly in the left posterior region. As for the second stage of number comparison, activation seemed to occur mainly in the right parieto–occipito–temporal junction. This finding is consistent with the results of a case study reported by Dehaene and Cohen (1997) in which a right parietal lesion caused problems in quantity estimation. Dehaene (1996) concluded his paper by noting that "the right hemisphere appears to possess both the ability to identify a digit and to represent its magnitude relative to other numbers" (p. 64).

The Neural Basis of Mathematical Ability

Perhaps the most controversial portion of the neuroscientific literature on math is the segment concerned with the neural basis of mathematical talent. To understand the origins of this controversy, we need to return to the bell-shaped (i.e., normal) distribution that was described earlier. Recall that in a normal distribution any given score falls into one of three categories: below average, average, or above average. Many years of research have shown that students always seem to fall into the same category (e.g., below average) each time they take a math test. Hence, there is a fair amount of stability over time in a student's performance as well as in his or her relative ranking in the distribution.

Although this pattern of results can be explained in a variety of ways (see Byrnes, 2001), advocates of the neural explanation of math talent (or NEMT, for short) suggest that there may be inborn differences in math ability that are reflected in distinct neural architectures. In the extreme, the NEMT perspective is reflected in the numerous attempts to reveal differences between Albert Einstein's brain and the brains of nongeniuses. Researchers who have done so have asked questions such as the following: Was his brain bigger? If so, in what areas of the brain were the differences in size most pronounced? Did he have more neurons of a particular type in particular layers of the cortex? Did he have more synaptic connections?

As I have suggested many times in this book, this atheoretical, bottom-up approach is not very efficient nor likely to be terribly informative. If math ability is like other kinds of abilities, it is likely to be comprised of a set of component skills that are carried out in specific regions of the brain. As such, two things have to occur before it even makes sense to look at structural or functional differences in brains: (1) psychologists have to create theories that carve math ability into component skills and (2) neuroscientists have to locate the brain regions responsible for carrying out these component skills. In the absence of such information, an individual could spend a great deal of time examining slices from brain regions that have nothing to do with math ability. In addition, most higher order skills are widely distributed throughout the brain (see Chapters 3, 4, and 6 for examples). Examination of slices of cortical tissue from one or two areas of the brain would not reveal the overall, brain-wide *organization* or neural architecture of a skill like math ability.

Third, there are two basic kinds of psychological theories: (1) those that merely subdivide a process into its component operations and (2) those that describe how the components should operate to produce *high levels* of performance. To see the difference between these types of theories, it is useful to consider the following analogy involving automobiles. The first kind of theory is like the answer that would be given to the question "How does a car engine work?" Here, one merely says what the component parts and processes are (e.g., "A *battery* sends a charge to a set of *spark plugs* that make sparks inside a set of *cylinders*. At the same time, *fuel injectors* spray atomized *gas* into the cylinders. . . . "); The second kind of theory, in contrast, would be more like the answer given to the question "Why is a race car faster than a family car?" Here, one elaborates on the basic description of components by referring to the *optimal* operation of the components and the system as a whole (e.g., faster cars have more cylinders, each of which permit a larger quantity of fuel to be ignited, etc.). Thus, a prerequisite for discovering possible differences in the brains of high-ability and low-ability students is a psychological theory that specifies the nature of mathematical *expertise* or talent. It is not enough to simply list the component operations of math skills. Once the optimal operation of the components has been defined, one can then consider how particular kinds of neural assemblies could support this optimal performance. For example, if one element of a theory of math ability suggests that math experts *quickly* retrieve facts, procedures, and strategies that are *relevant* to a given problem (e.g., Byrnes & Takahira, 1994), a neuroscientific approach would then attempt to consider possible brain architectures that would permit rapid, but selective, retrieval of problem-relevant information. A less informative approach would be to look for brain regions that seem to be active when math knowledge is retrieved. Such an approach is uninformative because it may not help a scientist discriminate among three kinds of people: (1) those who tend to retrieve relevant information, but do so fairly slowly; (2) those who tend to retrieve relevant information quickly; and (3) those who tend to retrieve irrelevant information quickly. It is conceivable that the same region of the brain could be active in all three types of individuals.

A fourth complicating issue pertains to the difference between *natural* ability (aptitude) and *acquired* expertise. Most advocates of the NEMT tend to focus on architectural differences that are alleged to be present *before* children have experiences that promote math knowledge. In other words, these advocates assume that the initial state of brain organization (or neural functioning) determines the manner in which mathematical knowledge and skill is acquired and utilized. One might argue, for example, that some students have more neurons in their frontal and parietal lobes that are available for being configured into performance-enhancing neural assemblies. Or one could argue that the process of myelination occurs more quickly in some people than in others. If so, then exposure to the same content in math class would not necessarily lead to the creation of similar kinds of neural assemblies in two individuals who are exposed to this content.

In contrast, the acquired expertise explanation would not focus on the initial differences in brain assemblies in people as much as differences that arise much later in development after formative experiences have transpired. Here, advocates of the latter position would agree that math experts probably have different brains than their less competent peers, but they would argue that experts have different brains because they have had experiences that nonexperts did not have. These experiences, in turn, helped to create appropriate neural assemblies (see Chapter 2 for more on how experience can sculpt brains in this way). Returning to the car analogy, then, the natural ability view would suggest that some people are born with "race cars" for brains while others are born with "family cars." The acquired expertise view, in contrast, would suggest that we all start off with "family cars" but some of us transform these cars into "race cars" through experience.

With all of these introductory comments in mind, we can now turn to several recent proposals regarding the origins of extreme mathematical talent (and gender differences in this regard). In an effort to understand the nature of giftedness, researchers at several universities in the United States have created summer programs to enhance the math skills of gifted seventh graders. In such programs, children are initially identified and selected on the basis of their very high standardized test scores in math or other subject areas. Once enrolled in a particular program, children are given a variety of tests, including the SATs. Remarkably, some of these children (less than 1%) have been found to score over 700 on the SAT (Benbow, 1988). This is quite a feat considering the fact that only 6% of much older students (i.e., twelfth graders) normally score that high. Moreover, further analyses showed that nearly all of the seventh graders who scored above 700 were male (the ratio is actually 12 males to every 1 female).

Confronted with such findings, it seems reasonable to ask two questions: (1) How is it possible for 13-year-olds to perform so well on a math test that is difficult for even twelfth graders (i.e., the SAT)? and (2) Why are gifted males more likely than gifted females to score above 700 on the SAT? Several different proposals have been advanced to explain these outcomes (Byrnes, 2001), but the explanation that has generated the most interest suggests that mathematical talent has a neural basis (see, e.g., Benbow, 1988, and commentaries). This NEMT begins by showing how gifted males and gifted females do not differ in their attitudes toward math. Moreover, their parents do not appear to hold sexist attitudes regarding math. Finally, these students have not attended high school, so a researcher could not argue that gender differences in extreme talent are due to the fact that males tend to take more high school math courses than females.

Inasmuch as various alternative explanations seemed to be inadequate, advocates of the NEMT began searching for evidence of possible anatomical or physiological indicators of math skill. They eventually found what they needed in the work of the late Norman Geschwind and colleagues on the anatomical basis of dyslexia. As I noted in Chapter 6, Geschwind et al. sought to account for three sets of findings: (1) a higher incidence of language problems in boys than in girls, (2) symmetry or reversed asymmetry in the size of certain brain areas in dyslexic children, and (3) unexpected empirical links between left-handedness, language disorders, and immune disorders (Geschwind & Behan, 1982; Geschwind & Galaburda, 1985). To explain all these findings, Geschwind and colleagues proposed the following. During prenatal development, testosterone levels affect the growth of the left cerebral hemisphere in such a way that an anomalous form of dominance develops. Instead of being right-handed and having language lateralized in the left hemisphere, affected individuals become left-handed with language lateralized in the right or both hemispheres. This altered physiology, in turn, leads to problems such as developmental dyslexia, impaired language development, and autism. Testosterone levels also affect the thymus, resulting in disorders of the immune system (e.g., allergies, colitis, AIDS). To explain asymmetries in the size of the left and right hemispheres, Geschwind and colleagues suggested the testosterone may either retard the growth of the left hemisphere or interfere with normal reductions in the right.

This proposal seemed promising to advocates of the NEMT because of the claim that some individuals might be born with atypical dominance and a larger-than-normal right hemisphere (Benbow, 1988). The reasoning was that "the right hemisphere is traditionally considered specialized for non-verbal tasks and the left for verbal, although these differences may not be qualitative but quantitative. Mathematical reasoning ability, especially in contrast to computational ability, may be more strongly under the influence of the right hemisphere" (Benbow, 1988, p. 180).

To test these speculations, Benbow and colleagues considered whether gifted children were more likely than nongifted children to be left-handed and to have immune disorders (e.g., allergies). To assess handedness, Benbow and colleagues gave the Edinburgh Handedness Inventory (Oldfield, 1971) to two kinds of children who were drawn from their sample of over 100,000 gifted students: (1) an extremely precocious group of children (N = 303) who scored above 700 on the SAT–math or above 630 on the SAT–verbal, and (2) a less precocious group who scored closer to 500 on the SAT–math (N = 127). Whereas the norms for Edinburgh Handedness Inventory suggest that 8% of Scottish adults use their left hands occasionally or often to perform everyday tasks, 13% of children who were extremely precocious for math and 10% of the less precocious group were left-handed in this way (Benbow, 1986). Whereas the incidence of left-handedness was found to be significantly higher in the extremely precocious children than in the Scottish adults (p < .04), two other comparisons revealed no significant differences: (1) less precocious children versus the Scottish adults and (2) extremely precocious children versus less precocious children. Note that the significant difference between the extremely precocious students and Scottish adults is largely a function of sample size. The adult sample contained over 1,000 adults. Had it contained as few as 600 individuals, the difference between 13% and 8% would no longer be significant.

As for gender differences in the extent of left-handedness in extremely precocious students, Benbow (1988) reports that more males (16%) than females (11%) were left-handed in the study ($p < .05$, using an unspecified test). However, the present author applied the standard test for comparing frequencies (i.e., the chi-square test) to Benbow's (1986) data and found that the difference between 16% and 11% is not significant ($p = .17$). In addition, the key difference between mathematically precocious males (14%) and mathematically precocious females (6%) was also not significant ($p = .33$).

With respect to immune disorders, Benbow (1988) reports that students with extremely high mathematical ability are twice as likely to have allergies as children in the general population (53% vs. 25%), but no statistical tests were employed in this instance presumably because the population figure was an estimate provided to Benbow by the author of the test for immune disorders. Such a difference would, however, be significant if the population rate of 25% were based on 10 or more children. A chi-square test applied to the percentages of extremely precocious students in math (53%) and less precocious students in the gifted sample (35%) revealed a highly significant difference ($p < .001$). As for extremely precocious males (53%) and females (54%), the difference in the incidence of allergies was not significant.

Thus, the preliminary findings based on handedness and allergies were not terribly supportive of the idea of greater right hemisphere involvement in gifted children, in general, and in gifted males, in particular. It could be argued, however, that these studies really do not test the right-hemisphere (RH) proposal directly because indices such as handedness and allergies are fairly imprecise. A more direct approach would be to look at patterns of activation in the right and left hemisphere using either neuroimaging or gross electrical recording techniques. In their review of the literature using the latter, O'Boyle and Gill (1998) report that gifted adolescents appear to engage their right hemispheres more than nongifted adolescents when they listen to auditory stimuli or process facial expressions. In addition, gifted adolescents show a pattern of resting activation that is similar to that of college students and significantly different from nongifted adolescents (i.e., greater activation in the frontal and occipital lobes).

Finally, comparisons of gifted males and females have revealed gender differences with respect to the involvement of the right hemisphere for the processing of faces and mental rotation (more involvement for males), but not for verbal stimuli. In addition, charts presented in Alexander, O'Boyle and Benbow (1996) also suggest greater resting activations in the parietal and possibly frontal lobes in gifted males than in gifted females, but these specific comparisons were not reported in the text. The one study that had the potential to consider whether greater right hemisphere involvement was associated with higher SAT–math scores (i.e., O'Boyle & Benbow, 1990) failed to report this correlation because the authors expressed concerns over a restricted range problem with the SAT–math scores (i.e., most students scored over 500). The authors did report a correlation of $r = -.29$ between laterality scores and SAT scores, but it was not clear from the text whether total SAT scores or just SAT–verbal scores were used to compute this correlation.

Thus, there is very little evidence in support of the idea that gifted children, in general, and gifted males, in particular, are better in math because they tend to engage their right hemispheres more than other individuals. In addition, there are other reasons to have serious doubts about this RH proposal. First, most neuroscientists assume that the frontal lobes are the most likely sites of higher order reasoning (Luria, 1973). More posterior regions of the right hemisphere could be associated with certain aspects of conceptual knowledge in math or certain types of spatial reasoning (but not all), but these regions are also active when working memory and attention are engaged (see Chapter 3). Thus, even if evidence suddenly did accumulate that suggested that extremely talented mathematicians engage their right hemispheres more than less talented individuals, this difference could reflect the former's greater reliance on math concepts, spatial skills, or working memory. These capacities may relate to the kind of reasoning required to do well on the SAT, but the core processes of problem comprehension and strategic planning are likely to be associated with the frontal lobes.

Second, it is not at all clear why a theory designed to account for reading disabilities (i.e., the model of Geschwind and colleagues) would even be appropriate for explaining high levels of math *talent*. If the Geschwind model really did apply, one would expect to find reading disabilities in many of the extremely precocious children. In fact, however, most of these children have a great deal of verbal ability in addition to having considerable math ability (Benbow, 1986, 1988). Third, in Chapter 6, it was noted that there is a very little evidence in support of the proposals of Geschwind and colleagues.

Fourth, advocates of the neural account have never really shown how knowledge-based or experience-based explanations are not viable. For example, whereas it is true that 13-year-olds tend not to take high school math courses, these children must get their knowledge and reasoning skills somewhere. Note that tests like the SAT–math require knowledge of arithmetic, algebra, and geometry. Many nongifted children receive direct instruction on these topics by the seventh or eighth grade, and most gifted children receive instruction on these topics 2 or more years before that. In addition, gifted children's enrichment in school involves exercises in problem-solving games and the like and they undoubtably pursue math-related activities outside of school as well. The only alternative to such an experience-based view is some form of radical nativism (i.e., these children did not need to be exposed to arithmetic, algebra, or geometry because they were born with knowledge of these topics). Thus, the question is not whether they have more knowledge than their nongifted peers, but how they learned it before their peers did.

Finally, it is worth noting that researchers may eventually find subtle, but important, architectural differences between the brains of gifted and nongifted children. What can be made of such differences if they are found? The arguments presented so far suggest the answer to this question is "very little." The key issue is not whether such differences exist but *how* and *when* they arose. Regarding the "how" aspect, the research presented in this book suggests that there are a number of factors that affect brain structure (e.g., genetics, hormones, and experience). With respect to the "when" aspect, note that some accounts claim that differences in brain structure exist prior to exposure to math content (the natural ability view), while others assume that differences arise in response to differential exposure to content (the acquired expertise view).

Summary of the Neuroscientific Literature

As can be surmised from the present chapter, there seem to be very few neuroscientific studies of math skills. As such, it is difficult to draw firm conclusions from this literature. What we can tentatively say is that (1) calculation skills seem to be largely confined to the left hemisphere (though not always); (2) individual math facts and procedures seemed to be stored in their own, separate areas of the cortex (e.g., one area for multiplication facts, another for subtraction procedures, etc.); (3) comparison and ordinality skills seem to be localized in the posterior regions of the right hemisphere (though not always); and (4) gifted children tend to have more allergies and engage their right hemisphere more often than nongifted children (though not always). There is, then, much to learn about the neuroscientific basis of math skills.

CONCLUSIONS, CAVEATS, AND
INSTRUCTIONAL IMPLICATIONS

Following the format I used in other chapters, I will address the implications of the research on math ability through a consideration of four questions:

1. How much overlap is there between the psychological and neuroscientific accounts of math skills?
2. Is it possible to fuse these accounts into a single integrated perspective?
3. How confident can we be in the portrait of math ability that has emerged from these two traditions?
4. When and how should children be taught math skills, given what we have learned from these two traditions?

The Overlap Question

Comparison of the psychological and neuroscientific perspectives on math ability suggests that these perspectives overlap very little. Whereas psychologists (and educators) have tended to emphasize multiple kinds of knowledge, strategies, and problem-solving skills, neuroscientists have tended to emphasize fairly low-level skills such as arithmetic calculation or ordinal judgments. Moreover, there is little indication that neuroscientists have used psychological accounts as "road maps" to help them locate regions of the brain that are responsible for performing the core operations of mathematical reasoning. Relatedly, it would appear that neuroscientific studies of math have had very little impact on contemporary psychological theories.

The reasons for this lack of overlap are not entirely clear, but two explanations seem plausible. The first is that relatively few neuroscientific studies of math have been conducted. Moreover, these studies are hard to find and easily missed. The second explanation is that math-specific deficits may be less common than language-specific, attention-specific, or memory-specific deficits (Dehaene, 1996). In other words, many of the people who experience math deficits also experience deficits in other domains. Individuals with such comorbidities seem to have been overlooked in the literature in favor of much rarer cases of "pure" acalculias. The greater preponderance of mixed disorders suggests that higher level performance in math may require the recruitment of important domain-general capacities such as working memory and a tendency to plan. The latter processes have been alleged to be centered in the frontal lobes (Luria, 1973; see Chapter 3 as well).

There is, however, a sense in which the psychological and neuroscientific perspectives can be said to overlap. In particular, the intriguing cases of double dissociations in math (see above) strongly support the assertions of psychologists and educators regarding the distinctions among declarative, conceptual, and procedural knowledge in math (Byrnes & Fox, 1998). Unfortunately, however, the same findings have little bearing on proposals regarding the possible links among these kinds of knowledge. Logically, at least three possibilities exist. The first is that math experts have all of the requisite knowledge (i.e., declarative, conceptual, and procedural) but this knowledge is not intrinsically interconnected. Instead, goal-related thinking and metacognitive processes search out the needed information (and strategies) and put these unconnected elements together. The second possible link is that high levels of conceptual knowledge help a student avoid procedural errors (Hiebert & LeFevre, 1987). The third is that conceptual knowledge serves as a foundation for learning procedures and also enhances motivation. Motivation is enhanced because students seem to be more attracted to content when it makes sense than when it does not make sense. The available brain research cannot be used to decide among these perspectives, and it is not clear whether brain research ever could.

The Integration Question

The constructs of "overlap" and "integration" are based on paradigms analogous to Venn diagrams or Hegel's discussion of thesis, antithesis, and synthesis. In the typical case (e.g., two competing theories), there are portions of the integrated quantities that overlap and portions that do not. In the case of the psychological and neuroscientific perspectives on math, however, the neuroscientific perspective is essentially subsumed by the psychological perspective with the exception of some specification of the brain areas that may be related to calculation and ordinal judgments. Hence, the psychological account has nearly everything the neuroscientific account has, and elaborates on this basic proposal considerably. As such, the simple answer to the question "Is it possible to fuse the psychological and neuroscientific perspectives into a single integrated perspective" is "Yes."

The Confidence Question

As I noted in other chapters, the confidence question hinges on two primary aspects of psychological and neuroscientific research: (1) the validity of the measures used and (2) the consistency of the results across studies. Applied to math research, the first issue is whether the measurement techniques used (e.g., paper-and-pencil tasks, EEG recordings, etc.) are valid indicators of math skills. A measure is valid to the extent that it assesses what you think it assesses (i.e., you think it measures X and it really does). Nonvalid measures, in contrast, are either misleading (i.e., we think it measures X but it really measures Y) or equivocal (i.e., a response could mean either X or mean Y). The consistency issue pertains to whether researchers in the psychological and neuroscientific camps have repeatedly found the same thing.

A comprehensive discussion of the validity and consistency of psychological research on math is beyond the scope of this chapter. It suffices to say that the research has been fairly consistent across studies, though controversies remain about such things as age trends (e.g., When do children first understand addition?) and the need to posit multiple forms of knowledge (e.g., conceptual, procedural, and declarative knowledge). For example, when we ask children to compute the answer to "0.35 + 2.19," is this task a measure of procedural knowledge or of other kinds of knowledge as well (e.g., conceptual knowledge)? Similarly, when we ask children to explain why $\frac{5}{6}$ is the answer to "$\frac{1}{2} + \frac{1}{3}$," is it accurate to say that they only rely on their conceptual knowledge when they provide an explanation? Even so, there is a growing consensus regarding the merits of the psychological description that was presented at the beginning of this chapter. In effect, psychologists and educators are reasonably confident that this description is accurate.

In contrast, it is far too early to be confident in the results of the neuroscientific studies described in this chapter. As I noted in Chapter 1, all neuroscientific methods have their problems. As result, we cannot feel confident about neuroscientific claims about math skills until multiple researchers find the same thing using different methods (e.g., case studies, PET, fMRI, EEG, and computer simulations). Thus, there is a real need for additional neuroscientific studies of math skills. Ideally, these new studies should be grounded in the description of mathematical talent that has emerged from the field of psychology. It would also be useful to begin to explore the architectures that would support superior levels of performance. Clues to the macrostructure of such an architecture could come from fMRI studies of gifted and nongifted children as they solve SAT-like problems. Once the active brain regions are revealed, researchers can then consider within-region and across-region microstructures that could support fast, accurate, and creative mathematical reasoning.

Instructional Implications

The preceding section can be summarized as follows: whereas we can be reasonably confident about the portrait of math skills that has emerged from the field of psychology, we cannot yet be confident about the math-related claims made by neuroscientists. As such, it would be most prudent to base all instructional implications on the psychological perspective (at least until more neuroscientific studies are conducted). Byrnes (2001) reviewed the extensive literature on the development of math skills and suggested the following implications:

1. Preschool experiences should be structured in such a way to enhance children's existing mathematical conceptual and procedural knowledge (however informal or implicit this knowledge may be). In other words, there is no need to wait until the first grade to have children begin to interact with mathematical ideas.
2. Instruction should form bridges between children's informal math ideas and the formal mathematics presented in school.
3. Instruction at all levels should be consistent with the "Math 2000" recommendations of the National Council of Teachers of Mathematics (1998). The consensus view of math skills that was presented earlier serves as a foundation for many of these recommendations.
4. Instructional activities should promote the acquisition of number concepts as well as schemata for various kinds of word problems. One of the best ways to instill such knowledge in students is to have them solve structurally similar problems and consider how these problems are similar (Gick & Holyoak, 1983; Sweller & Cooper, 1985).
5. Exercises should be designed to promote an accurate metacognitive understanding of when an answer is sensible and correct, and when it is not.
6. Finally, there is no substitute for extensive practice. Even when teachers tie procedures to concrete referents or rely on meaningful problem solving, students still make a variety of procedural errors (Byrnes, 1992; Peterson, Carpenter, Fennema, & Loef, 1989; Resnick & Omanson, 1987). Although there is no dichotomy between "meaning," on the one hand, and "repetition," on the other, many people often assume there is. The best approach involves embedding practice within meaningful, goal-directed activities.

CHAPTER 8

Conclusions

In the present chapter, my goal is to revisit, integrate, and discuss the implications of the research and arguments that I have presented so far. A useful way to approach this task is to address the following two questions: (1) How could brain research be relevant to psychological theory and educational practice? and (2) What have we learned from psychologically relevant and educationally relevant brain research and what do we still need to know? The first part of this chapter is devoted to answering these two questions. In the second part, my goal is to evaluate some of the claims about the brain that have appeared in the popular press, practitioner-oriented publications, and parent-oriented publications in recent years.

THE EDUCATIONAL AND PSYCHOLOGICAL RELEVANCE
OF BRAIN RESEARCH: KNOWNS AND UNKNOWNS

Readers of this book have probably encountered the concept of relevance if they have ever conducted web-based searches for specific kinds of information. In such searches, first one enters a keyword or several keywords into a search engine (e.g., "common cold remedies") and then the search engine generates a list of web pages that are alleged (by the search engine) to be relevant to this domain. A scan of the list usually reveals, however, that some sites are relevant (e.g., a health-related site with information on common colds), while others are not (e.g., a site that has information on what to do when a common law marriage turns "cold"). For obvious reasons, one only searches further in the former kind of sites because only they can help provide the desired information.

As this example illustrates, people usually judge information to be relevant to the extent that it helps them accomplish their goals (Pintrich & Schunk, 1996). As such, one would expect that psychologists would only try to learn more about the brain if they believed that this exercise would help them accomplish their professional goals of learning more about the mind or learning more about development. Similarly, one would expect that educators would only try to learn more about the brain if they believed that this exercise would help them accomplish their professional goals of learning more about effective forms of instruction or understanding students better. The present book was written to show how brain research can be used to foster a better understanding of the mind, development, and effective instructional practices—if this research is approached in a particular way.

As I noted in earlier chapters, this "particular way" pertains to the fact that psychological theories carve the mind into different components and subcomponents (e.g., long-term vs. short-term memory). If there were only one way to carve up a given psychological function or skill (e.g., memory), there would be no need to conduct experiments. It is the case, however, that there are quite a number of ways to decompose psychological functions into their constituents. In addition, there are quite a number of ways to explain development. To decide among these possibilities, psychologists need to conduct experiments to "rule in" certain models and "rule out" others. It has been argued in this book and elsewhere (e.g., Kosslyn & Koenig, 1992) that the data from traditional psychological experiments should be combined with data from neuroscientific studies to bolster the claims of a particular theoretical account. Over time, it is hoped that these collective efforts would lead to the development of highly accurate theories of psychological processes.

The most important consequence of developing more accurate theories of mental processes would be that these theories would constitute the conceptual basis of more effective forms of instruction (the latter being a form of procedural knowledge). Whereas effective forms of instruction are compatible with the design of the mind, ineffective forms are incompatible with this design (Byrnes, 2001). Hence, just as math procedures are more likely to be used appropriately if a student has accurate mathematical conceptual knowledge (see Chapter 7), instructional techniques are more likely to be used appropriately if a teacher has accurate conceptual knowledge of student learning, student behavior, cognitive development, and motivation.

The foregoing analysis implies that brain research is only relevant to the fields of psychology and education to the extent that it helps foster a more accurate understanding of the mind, development, and learning. Whereas some aspects of brain research are likely to foster such an improved understanding, other aspects are not likely to do so because they are several steps removed from direct applications. Consider, for example, the following two items of information that one could glean from the neuroscientific literature: (1) there seem to be separate brain areas for verbal and spatial working memory (see Chapter 3), and (2) neuronal impulses rely on the flow of potassium ions. Whereas the former item would be directly relevant to the goals of psychologists and educators, the latter would only be indirectly relevant at best. For efficiency's sake, then, it would seem that psychologists and educators should only make the effort to become familiar with the former kinds of information.

Having discussed the issue of how brain research could be relevant, I can now consider the implications of some of the findings that *are* relevant (according to the criteria set out here). In Chapter 2, on brain development, we learned that there are two primary kinds of processes that determine the brain's initial and later cytoarchitecture: intrinsic and extrinsic. The *intrinsic* factors are determined by genetic instructions and include such things as (1) the number, type, and eventual location of cells in different parts of the brain; (2) the projection of axons to particular targets; and (3) the spontaneous firing of neurons to promote "preexperience" patterns of interconnections. The *extrinsic* factors include such things as afferent stimulation (e.g., visual and other kinds of experiences), competition among neurons for trophic factors, chemical signals among neighboring neurons, nutrition, and toxins. At the very least, this account suggests that the neural organization of an adult brain is not set in stone at birth. In addition, it suggests that there are many ways to explain a structural difference that might emerge over time between the brains of two individuals (e.g., genetics, experience, prenatal nutrition, etc.). As such, it would be unwise to retroactively reason back from an observed brain difference to one particular factor (without corroborative evidence). For example, if genes, experience, and nutrition could all cause a structural difference that might someday be observed in postmortem studies of men and women (e.g., a higher density of neurons in the right parietal lobe), it would be inappropriate to assume that this difference must have been caused by genes (because it could have also been caused by experience or nutrition).

In Chapter 3, on memory, we learned that (1) memory is a multifaceted process that is widely distributed across the brain, and (2) there is a fair amount of overlap between the psychological and neuroscientific views of memory. Regarding the latter point, it can be said that memory research might be the paradigmatic example of how psychologists and neuroscientists could work together to develop a dovetailing perspective.

For example, psychologists forged some of their theoretical distinctions (e.g., implicit vs. explicit memory) partly on the basis of studies of brain-injured patients. Neuroscientists, for their part, have regularly used psychological theories of memory as roadmaps to find memory-specific regions of the brain. This is not to say, however, that everything has been worked out in the field of memory. There still is a great deal of slippage among individual studies (e.g., conflicting findings regarding the locations of putative memory sites in the brain) and there are a number of topics that have inspired heated debates that are still unresolved (e.g., the phenomenon of long-term potentiation). Thus, a great deal of additional work needs to be done to verify and refine an integrated view of memory. A particularly important line of work would be to understand the biological basis of phenomena like consolidation and the formation of the neural assemblies that underlie memory records.

In Chapter 4, on attention, we learned that attention seems to consist of an orienting network, an executive network, and a vigilance network. These networks are primarily associated with certain regions of both parietal lobes, the right frontal lobe, and the anterior cingulate gyrus. In addition, we learned that there are certain tracts of dopaminergic and noradrenergic neurons that may relate to arousal, and that flashbulb memories may arise from the interplay of adrenal hormones, enhanced glucose in the blood, and focused attention. Unlike the memory field, in which neuroscience and psychology seem to have contributed equally to an integrated view, the attention literature seems to be largely dominated by the psychological perspective (particularly the viewpoints of cognitive, developmental, and clinical psychologists). Thus, it would seem that an infusion of neuroscientific studies is needed to refine and extend the psychological perspective. In addition, more work is needed to understand the neuroscientific basis of attention deficit disorders and the inverted-U-shaped developmental curve for certain attentional processes (i.e., improvement from infancy to middle childhood, stable performance through late adulthood, declining performance in old age). Moreover, there is no apparent consensus on the region(s) of the brain that might be responsible for the selectivity of attention. Is it the thalamus? The lateral geniculate nucleus? The locus ceruleus?

In Chapter 5, on emotions, we learned that the psychological and neuroscientific perspectives on this topic do not overlap very much. To illustrate, various psychological theories suggest that emotions involve both an appraisal component and a response component. Relatively few neuroscientists have attempted to locate regions of the brain that are active when either of these two components are engaged. Similarly, a lot of neuroscientific work is directed at understanding the neuroanatomy of fear, but this work has had little bearing on contemporary psychological theories of fear (or psychological theories of emotion in general). This lack-of-influence problem has been further complicated by the fact that a number of inconsistencies have arisen in neuroscientific studies of emotion. Thus, it is not yet possible to derive an integrative view of emotion from the available psychological and neuroscientific research (Davidson & Ekman, 1994; LeDoux, 1995). One way to foster the development of such a view would be to encourage emotion researchers to follow the example of their colleagues in the field of memory. Another positive development would be for researchers in the motivation area to join forces with psychologists and neuroscientists who study emotion. Such a move would help emotion research to have more of an impact on instructional practices than it currently has.

In Chapter 6, on reading, we learned that the psychological and neuroscientific research on reading supports two main conclusions. The first is that reading consists of multiple tasks that are performed in concert. For example, there are processes related to (1) perceiving letters and groups of letters, (2) pronunciation of letter and word strings, (3) syntactic processing related to function words (e.g., "or") and word endings (e.g., "-ing"), (4) semantic processes related to retrieving word endings, and (5) conceptual processes related to the abstract–concrete continuum. The second conclusion is that these processes seem to be at least weakly modular and redundant. At a general level, then, the psychological and neuroscientific perspectives on reading seem to overlap and converge on a common understanding. At a more specific level, however, the research on topics such as the neuroscientific basis of reading disabilities, precocious readers, and reading readiness is not very conclusive. Moreover, there is still work to be done to determine the precise locations and component operations of the four processors shown in Figure 6.1, and to see whether this model needs to be elaborated. By resolving these issues in additional research, we will develop more accurate models of reading. These models, in turn, will have direct implications for instructional practice.

In Chapter 7, on math, we learned that psychological descriptions of mathematical ability have tended to be more elaborate than neuroscientific accounts. Relatedly, psychologists and educators have been much more likely than neuroscientists to conduct studies of math performance. Despite these discrepancies, however, the evidence as a whole supports the distinctions among declarative, procedural, and conceptual knowledge in math that have been argued for by psychologists and educators. Moreover, interesting double dissociations have emerged from case studies of brain-injured individuals. In the future, it is hoped that neuroscientists will use the more elaborate psychological models of math skills as guides to find possible regions of brain activity for the components of math ability. In addition, it is hoped that researchers will come to a better understanding of the neuroanatomical basis of mathematical disabilities and extreme mathematical talent. The latter outcomes would have enormous implications for instructional practice and for our understanding of the origins and nature of gender differences in math skills.

Overall, then, it has been shown that researchers in certain fields (e.g., memory, reading) are well ahead of their colleagues in other fields (e.g., emotion, math) in terms of their tendency to integrate the psychological and neuroscientific perspectives on some topic of interest. In addition, we have seen that there are still a number of fundamental questions and issues that have yet to be addressed. These questions and issues include the following:

1. We know that genetics and epigenetic processes work together to sculpt a person's brain. To what extent are the epigenetic influences constrained by genetics? In other words, is it possible to overcome a genetic predisposition (e.g., to have reading problems) if epigenetic processes are especially favorable? Conversely, is it possible for problems to arise even when there is no genetic predisposition?

2. What exactly does it mean for the brain to be ready to learn something?

3. Macrolevel comparisons of the brains of (a) men and women, (b) gifted and nongifted children, (c) Einstein and the rest of us, and (d) reading-disabled and nondisabled people have failed to reveal any obvious or consistent differences in terms of such things as the relative size of particular regions, the shape of these regions, or the number of neurons in each region. What kinds of brains (or brain regions) could support a high level or a low level of performance in any given domain? How are these brains (or brain regions) formed?

4. How does the brain represent a piece of information as a neural assembly? How are these assemblies created through experience? How long does it take to create an assembly (or permanent record)? How many times do neurons have to fire together to form a stable assembly?

5. How exactly are flashbulb memories created?

6. Are there regions of the brain (other than the amygdala) that are specifically devoted to emotional processing?

7. The links between mind and brain seem to be probabilistic. For example, studies show that brain regions that are supposedly responsible for specific skills (e.g., subtraction) are sometimes inactive when the skill

is being expressed by an individual. How could this be? Relatedly, how could damage to different regions of the cortex produce the same deficit?

The existence of such fundamental questions suggests that we still have a long way to go before we can fully understand the relationship between the mind and the brain. Other complications become apparent when one compiles all the facts about brain regions that were discussed in Chapters 3 through 7. The frontal lobes, for example, have been found to be associated with all of the following: word finding, episodic memory, verbal working memory, interference, memory strategies, meta-memory, attentional vigilance, stress, arousal, inhibition, processing emotional facial expressions, semantic associates of emotions, sustained emotional context, depression, positive and negative emotions, reading words, defining words, rhyming, and higher order reasoning. The temporal lobes, in contrast, have been found to be associated with all of the following: processing and storage of auditory and phonological information, declarative memory, consolidation, recall, recognition, semantic memory, the epigastric sensation in emotions, emotional processing, and acquired dyslexia. The parietal lobes have been found to be associated with spatial working memory, episodic memory, three aspects of attention (disengaging, orienting, and vigilance), and neglect of the initial or final portions of words (when these lobes are damaged). Whereas the occipital lobes are only implicated in the processing of visually presented words and spatial working memory, the junctions of the occipital lobe and other lobes are implicated in the recognition of tools (bilateral occipital–temporal–parietal junctions), word recognition (left occipital–temporal–parietal junction), number comparison and magnitude code (bilateral occipital–temporal–parietal junction), visual arabic numbers (left occipital–temporal junction), and recognition of animals (bilateral medial occipital–ventral temporal junction). At the subcortical level, the striatum is associated with sensorimotor skills, arousal, depression, and the ability to recognize facial expressions of anger, fear, and disgust. The amygdala is associated with fear, stress, anger, and depression. Whereas the cerebellum is associated with classically conditioned motor responses, the thalamus is associated with rote memory, the filtering aspect of attention, arousal, fear conditioning, and depression.

When all of these findings are considered together, it would seem that any given region of the brain performs multiple tasks. If we just consider the Broca area of the left frontal lobe, for example, we see that it seems to be involved in word finding, reading words aloud, defining words, speech production, constructing syntactic relations during reading, verbal working memory, and depression. Although one could ex-

plain most of these findings by arguing for the existence of some unde-
fined capacity that underlies all verbal tasks, such a claim would not be
terribly informative nor could it explain the link to depression. When we
are confronted with this evidence, we have two options: (1) we can assume that all of these skills really are subserved by the Broca area and
then wonder why this might be the case (e.g., Posner & Raichle, 1994)
or (2) we can question whether these skills all are located in the Broca
area and think about alternative models in which given regions are more
like "way stations" than "homes" for skills. While we ponder such di-
lemmas, we can toss in several other unresolved issues regarding the
meaning of blood flow results (e.g., Is a brain region active when blood
is flowing to it or away from it?) and EEG recordings (e.g., Is increased
power a sign of greater or lesser activation?). Hence, it is difficult to be
smug or overly confident about many of the results reported in this
book. However, it would also be wrong to dismiss all of them out of
hand because, in a number of cases, the findings are consistent with
those from traditional experiments in psychology.

EVALUATING CLAIMS ABOUT THE BRAIN

As I noted in Chapter 1, brain research has taken on a life of its own in
the popular press and in teacher-oriented outlets (Bransford, Brown, &
Cocking, 1999). It seems that nearly every month, there is yet another issue of *Time* or *Newsweek* that has a focus on brain research. Moreover,
there seems to be no shortage of teacher-oriented books, companion vid-
eos, and articles on how a teacher can "teach to the brain" (e.g., Jensen,
1998; Sylwester, 1995). How accurate are the claims made in these outlets? In this final section, we will consider the extent to which some of
claims that have received the most attention follow from the available
neuroscientific research. The rationale for the present section is nicely
summarized by Wolfe and Brandt (1998, p. 10), who argue: "[Educa-
tors] need to critically read and analyze the research in order to separate
the wheat from the chaff. If educators do not develop a functional understanding of the brain and its processes, [they] will be vulnerable to
pseudoscientific fads, inappropriate generalizations, and dubious programs." Bransford et al. (1999) add: "Neuroscience has advanced to the
point where it is time to think critically about the form in which research
information is made available to educators so that it is interpreted appropriately for practice—identifying which research findings are ready
for implementation and which are not."

In the present book, it is assumed that the best way to critically read and analyze general-audience descriptions of brain research is to be familiar with (1) the kinds of errors that can be observed in these descriptions and (2) the protective measures that can be used to guard against falling prey to erroneous information. Three kinds of errors can be observed. The first can be called the "source incredulity error" because it has to do with the credibility of particular findings or the person being interviewed. To guard against this error, readers can adopt the stance of always "considering the source." The first thing to note in this regard is that certain scientific journals will publish just about anything, even if the study is inherently flawed. Thus, the simple fact that a finding has been published in a journal does not mean that it is valid, meaningful, or likely to be replicated. Second, sometimes an experimental finding in a journal is "significant" in the statistical sense, but trivial in a real-world sense. For example, a correlation of $r = .20$ might be significant if a study had 300 people in it, but the absolute size of this correlation is very small. Similarly, a group difference in IQ scores of, say, 4 points might be statistically significant but correspond to only a difference of maybe one additional correct answer on an IQ test (if that). Third, when reporters are unable to get interviews with the authors of a particular provocative study, they will also interview others who are familiar with the study and who ostensibly would be considered respectable sources by their readership (e.g., an author of a book such as this, anyone with a medical degree, etc.). Not that long ago there was an inverse relationship between being willing to talk to the press and knowing what you are talking about. In recent years, this phenomenon has changed somewhat, but one still has to be careful. Thus, the following questions need to be asked when evaluating the merits of a particular claim:

> Is this claim based on a well-designed study whose results were published in a journal with high standards?
> Has the study been replicated by others in independent labs?
> If so, is the reporter talking to the authors of these studies or to someone else?
> If it is someone else, is this person a credible source? (e.g., Does he or she regularly publish research articles on the same topic? Does he or she have a full-time appointment at a top-ranked university?).

Now let's say that a claim is based on findings that pass the tests above (i.e., the study was well designed and published in a respectable outlet; the interviewee is credible). The next kind of error is the "misinterpretation error," which is caused by a reporter or textbook author's misinterpretation of what he or she has heard during an interview or read. Having been interviewed by magazine and newspaper reporters several times myself, I am familiar with the tendency of reporters to either misunderstand the meaning of my results or to draw implications from my studies that just are not there (because the real implications are not as interesting to a wide audience as they had hoped!). Unfortunately, the only way to guard against this problem is to check out the accuracy of claims oneself by reading the original research. Most people, however, do not have the time, inclination, or expertise to validate the majority of neuroscientific claims.

Now let's assume that the source is credible and that no distortion of the original information has occurred. The third error might be called the "unwarranted inferential leaps error." In one kind of uwarranted inferential leap, either the expert being interviewed or the reporter doing the interviewing takes two or more credible findings and puts them together in ways that do not necessarily follow. The resultant claim is a speculation based on indirect strands of evidence, but the author writes as though the actual research that directly supports the claim has been done. To illustrate this phenomenon, it has been found (in credible research) that (1) the human brain has receptors for sex hormones and (2) autopsies of rat brains show sexual dimorphisms (e.g., larger corpus callosums in females). From these two findings, many experts assumed that there probably were sexual dimorphisms in human brains as well and freely supplied this information to the press (even though they had no direct evidence to support this in the case of human brains). When brain scans were eventually done on humans, however, these scans showed no evidence of obvious structural differences (see Chapter 2). The best way to guard against being mislead by such speculations is to ask "Has the actual study that supports this claim been done?"

A second kind of inferential leap comes when an author or expert says that a particular set of neuroscientific findings clearly support a particular psychological model or method of instruction, but forgot to mention (or did not realize) that these findings would also support a number of alternatives. To illustrate this problem, note that many scientists and parents have observed that young infants regularly insert things into their mouths. To explain this behavior, scientists at various times have argued that it reflects (1) children's tendency to understand the world by acting on it, (2) the fact that children have been reinforced for doing this sort of behavior (e.g., doing so with bottles yields milk), and (3) children get sexual gratification by doing so. The fact that the behavior is consistent with all three of these claims means that it does not unequivocally support any one of the them (i.e., it is ambiguous). The only way to guard against this problem is to critically ask whether a particular finding would only be consistent with a particular theory or instructional approach. In the case of instructional approaches, for example, the first step would be to think of a competing instructional strategy that people are currently using or used in the recent past. The second would be to consider whether the data would only be consistent with one of the two approaches.

In sum, then, the three primary kinds of errors include source incredulity errors, distortion errors, and unwarranted inferential leap errors. With these problems in mind, we can now turn to some of the claims that have recently appeared in the popular press, teacher-oriented publications, or parent-oriented publications. For efficiency's sake, the analysis will be limited to a small set of claims that have tended to appear in many of these outlets. In addition to showing problems with these claims, I hope to model the process by which one can interpret the evidence critically using the information in this book. As another space-saving measure, I will typically paraphrase each claim rather than provide actual quotes from articles or books.

Let's begin with the most general of the claims that appear in popular outlets:

Claim 1: Experience creates new synaptic connections among neurons and also alters existing patterns of connections.

From the information presented earlier in this book (e.g., Chapters 2 and 3), we can see that this claim is an accurate portrayal of a mainstream neuroscientific assumption. However, more specific versions of this claim do not fare so well. Consider, for example, the following suggestion:

Claim 1a: A child's brain will not work properly (or as well as it could) if it does not receive the right amount of stimulation at the right time.

To support this claim, various authors refer to so-called windows of opportunity for learning in the visual system, auditory system, and areas of the brain for music. In the visual system, for example, they describe findings involving animals with surgically closed eyelids or human infants with cataracts to show how exposure to visual information is required for the development of normal vision (Kosslyn & Koenig, 1994). In the auditory system, findings suggest that newborns lose the ability to discriminate between certain phonemes by their first birthday if these phonemes are not used in their native language (Kuhl, 1998), and other findings suggest that people who learn foreign languages after age 12 never seem to lose their accent. In music, it has been found (in a single study) that the movements involved in playing an instrument activate a specific area of the motor cortex, and that musicians who began their music training before age 10 showed a greater range of activation than those who received their training later (Elbert, Pantev, Wienbruch, Rockstroh, & Taub, 1995).

How might these findings be interpreted? To begin with, it can be noted that the articles in question pass the source credulity test because the findings were originally published in top journals and the key players were interviewed. However, whereas these findings are compelling, they probably have very little practical value. The visual and auditory research, for example, merely shows how Mother Nature decided that it would be better to use experience to finish the basic wiring for lower level sensory operations after birth than before birth (presumably to conserve energy). She bet that (1) most people would be born without cataracts, (2) most people would not have their eyelids sewn shut, and (3) their environments would have plenty of light and numerous objects to observe. All three expectations seem like pretty good bets (Bruer, 1998). Second, the skills that have clear windows of opportunity are associated with ubiquitious properties of the natural *physical* environment. There is little reason to think that evolution would have selected music and other cultural artifacts in the same way that it selected certain aspects of visual and auditory systems. Third, to show that a minimum amount of experience is required to get basic skills up and running is not to say that a *large* amount of experience during a window of opportunity will make someone into an *exceptional* performer. Fourth, vision and phonetic processing are complex processes that are made up of smaller component operations. Some of the smaller components have their own critical periods that occur well before or past the widely cited ones, while others have no critical period at all (Bruer, 1998). Hence, it makes little sense to speak of *a* critical period for vision or hearing. Finally, it is not clear how the findings regarding activated areas of the motor cortex in musicians is relevant to the issue of windows of opportunity. For example, the findings do not show that musicians trained after age 10 never attain high levels of skill. Instead, they simply show that skilled performers who received their training after age 10 activate a smaller area of the cortex. In addition, the literature on expertise demonstrates that it is not when one starts that matters as much as the amount of time spent in daily, deliberate practice (Ericsson, 1996). The minimum amount seems to be 3.5 hours of deliberate practice per day over

10 years. If so, then to attain a high level of skill by the time one reaches the typical age of entry into prestigious schools of music (e.g., 18), one would have to start before age 10.

Notwithstanding all these concerns, some authors have used the results regarding windows of opportunity to argue that parents need to "provide lots of sensory experiences—tasting, touching, seeing, hearing, and smelling. These experiences build the connections that build your child's brain" (Dodge & Heronman, 1999, p. 43). In a related way, authors of articles in education journals and the popular press have used the findings to argue that second language learning and music education need to begin during the preschool period (e.g., Begley, 1996; Jensen, 1998; Weinberger, 1998), before the windows of opportunity "slam shut." Based on the arguments above, these suggestions may be unwarranted inferential leaps. I would agree that second language learning and music education should start early, but I would not base my entire argument on brain research.

Two other experience-related claims have also found their way into the popular press, teacher-oriented publications, or parent-oriented publications (hereafter collectively called "publications for nonscientists"):

> *Claim 1b: Certain prenatal and postnatal experiences can alter the brain forever.*

and

> *Claim 1c: Experiences from one domain can create favorable brain structures that not only support good performance in that domain, but also support good performance in other domains.*

Let's begin with Claim 1b. Considerable attention has been given in publications for nonscientists to the effect that stress can have on brain development. In particular, various authors have argued that excessive levels of cortisol (a substance secreted by the adrenal glands during stress reactions) causes permanent damage to several regions of the brain, including the hippocampus (important for memory) and the locus ceruleus (important for selective attention). In support of this claim, they refer to three main lines of evidence. First, studies have shown that institutionalized children have smaller temporal structures than control children. Second, neuroimaging techniques have shown that adults diagnosed with posttraumatic stress disorder (PTSD) have smaller hippocampal areas than adults without the disorder (Bremner, 1999; Sapolsky, 1999). Third, children in high-risk environments have elevated levels of cortisol and also show cognitive and behavioral profiles consistent with the idea of problems in attention and memory (Gunnar & Barr, 1998).

To evaluate this evidence critically, it is helpful to ask two questions: (1) Is it reasonable to expect that cortisol could cause brain damage in these areas? And (2) Are there areas of uncertainty in the evidence that could cause one to view it with caution? Regarding the first question, it is reasonable to expect that cortisol could cause brain damage in these areas because these areas have receptors for cortisol (Sapolsky, 1999). Moreover, studies with animals suggest that size reductions do occur when high levels of cortisol are experimentally expressed into these areas (Sapolsky, 1999). Further, acute administrations of cortisol in humans cause temporary memory and attentional problems (e.g., Schmidt et al., 1999).

However, regarding the second question, there are also important areas of uncertainty in this research. For example, the hippocampus is one of the few brain regions that produces new neurons after birth and continues to do so well into old age (Sapolsky, 1999). If so, then it is not clear how a single, circumscribed period of trauma could cause permanent or irreversible damage to this structure. A recent study, in fact, showed that a reduction in cortisol can reverse hippocampal atrophy in patients who have a cortisol-related disorder (i.e., Starkman et al., 1999). This regeneration argument would be especially true for young children, who have been found to be remarkably plastic even after having large areas of their brains removed (see Chapter 2). Relatedly, it is not clear how one should interpret the evidence that traumatized individuals perform poorly on measures of memory and attention. Does this lower level of performance reflect the fact that their brains have been damaged by their earlier trauma or the fact that many of these individuals still have high levels of cortisol circulating in their blood?

Another problem pertains to the amount of cell loss that has to occur before cognitive problems ensue. Although the average man's brain is 9% larger than the average woman's brain, no gender differences have been found in male versus female intelligence levels. Some of the cortisol studies have found reductions that were smaller than 9%. Would such small reductions lead to cognitive problems? Finally, cell count methods have often been criticized for being biased. One source of bias is the fact that the person doing the counting is also the one looking for a reduction. A second kind occurs when researchers compare the raw cell count from one group (e.g., PTSD adults) to the raw cell count for another group (e.g., controls) instead of adjusting these counts by measures of total cortical volume in each individual (Sapolsky, 1999). A third problem is that pretrauma measures of cognition and attention are usually not administered because it is hard to anticipate the likely victims of trauma and give these individuals pretests. It is possible that group differences in cognition and attention existed prior to exposure to stress and this difference in ability means that the focal group may be more vulnerable to the effects of stress (Masten & Coatsworth, 1998; Sapolsky, 1999). Collectively, these areas of uncertainty reflect the problem of source incredulity error discussed earlier.

Using similar arguments, one can question a related kind of finding that was recently described in the September 27, 1999, issue of *Newsweek*: "Biologists reported on a study of people with asymmetries in traits like feet, fingers, ears and elbows. IQs were lower in asymmetric people by about as much (percent wise) as their measurements deviated from perfect symmetry. Some sort of stress during fetal development probably causes asymmetry. . . . The same stress may cause imperfections in the developing nervous system leading to less efficient neurons for sensing, remembering, and thinking." Apart from the fact that such a finding runs contrary to everything we know about the plasticity of infants, the article in question was based on a study published in a second-tier journal. Moreover, the correlation between asymmetry in hand size and IQ was a mere $r = -.24$ (more asymmetry, lower IQ score).

The blurb above came from a larger article on so-called fetal programming in which prenatal events are said to alter the physiology of fetuses (e.g., make them smaller). These alterations, in turn, are thought to make them more susceptible to diseases like diabetes and high blood pressure. As argued by Peter Nathanielsz (1999) in his book on fetal programming (*Life in the Womb: The Origin of Health and Disease*), "What happens to you in womb can program your health for a lifetime." Although the theory has really caught on in the field of epidemiology, there are many problems with the evidence that has accumulated to support it (Trafford, 1999). First, diseases are determined by a host of genetic and environmental factors. As such, there usually is no one culprit. Second, most of the associations between birth weight and outcomes are just that: associations. When two things co-occur, it does not follow that one necessarily causes the other. Moreover, these associations are fairly small (though often significant due to extremely large samples). Third, whereas low birth weight is related to higher rates of health problems, the vast majority of low-birth-weight infants lack these problems. Finally, the "womb doom" theory fails to acknowledge the remarkable ability of infants to be resistant to numerous kinds of insults (see Chapter 2).

Thus, Claim 1b (that certain experiences can alter the brain forever) is still open to question. What about Claim 1c, that experiences from one domain can create favorable brain structures that not only support good performance in that domain, but also support good performance in other domains? Let's begin our critique of this claim by considering three examples. In the literature for nonscientists, it has been suggested that music training not only improves musical skills, it also improves math skills and spatial skills. The authors explain such improvements by suggesting that (1) music training alters certain structures in the right hemisphere and (2) musical ability, math ability, and spatial ability all rely on these structures (Dodge & Heronman, 1999; Begley, 1996). As a second example, the literature suggests that physical activity not only promotes brain development in motor areas (e.g., the cerebellum and motor cortices), it also promotes brain development in other areas (Dodge & Heronman, 1999; Jensen, 1998; Sylwester, 1995). As a third example, the literature suggests that enriched environments create thicker cortices, larger cell bodies, and more extensive dendritic branching in the brain; these changes, in turn, subtend higher levels of intelligence and performance (Begley, 1996; Jensen, 1998).

To evaluate these findings, one can ask: (1) Are the findings credible?, (2) Did the authors misinterpret the findings?, and (3) Did the authors engage in unwarranted inferential leaps? It turns out that the findings are not very credible in the case of the music and physical activity examples. The music studies, for example, were published in journals with questionable standards. In addition, independent labs have repeatedly failed to replicate the results (e.g., Steele, Bass, & Crook, 1999). Further, in the most cited study (Rauscher et al., 1997), children either received piano lessons, computer keyboard work, or other kinds of activities. Whereas only those with piano lessons showed improved spatial skills, children were not randomly assigned to conditions. Parents were allowed to choose conditions and it is not clear how much they knew about the goals of the study. With respect to the alleged effects of physical activity, the authors failed to cite empirical studies to support their claims. Thus, advocates of music and physical education will have to turn to other avenues besides brain research to support their claim that these subject areas should be central to the curriculum (e.g., Jensen, 1998; Sylwester, 1995).

As for the third example regarding the effects of enriched environments on brain structure, the results are credible and well established. Moreover, the authors do not misinterpret the evidence in this regard.

They do, however, engage in a certain amount of unwarranted inference making. Whereas it is true that more complex environments lead to physical changes in rat brains, the changes are highly specific and localized to the cerebellar cortex (Kleim et al., 1998). Moreover, there is no evidence that these changes make the animals more "intelligent" (in the way that this term is usually applied to humans). In fact, there is good reason to think that cognitive development sometimes involves a "distillation" of a more streamlined macrostructure out of more elaborate, detailed structures. Hence, "more" is not always better. In essence, then, whereas we can be sure that complex environments alter brain structures, we still have no idea how to manipulate this process to children's advantage (Bransford et al., 1999; Bruer, 1998). Would it be better to spend a long time on a few "big ideas" in science or history, or go over lots of smaller ideas? Which environment is more complex? Would either approach alter the brain for the better?

The final claim to be discussed is the following:

Claim 2: Brain research validates long-held principles of effective teaching.

In teacher-oriented publications, several authors have alleged that brain research is consistent with the principles of constructivist teaching, the importance of meaningful instruction, and even Madeline Hunter's Mastery Teaching approach (Caine & Caine, 1997; Lowery, 1998; Wolfe, 1998). To support constructivism, they argue that the brain must take widely distributed information from several modalities and put it all together when thinking occurs. While this is true, several decidedly nonconstructivist approaches also suggest that this kind of information integration must occur (e.g., connectionism). To support the importance of meaning, they argue that the brain is a meaning-making organ that is also inherently social. As I noted in Chapter 1, however, meaning resides in the domain of psychology, not biology. There is nothing in a neural connection that makes it meaningful. To support Hunter's approach, research on procedural memory, task analysis, and rehearsal are described. However, it is not clear how this research is neuroscientific. It is more properly viewed as traditionally psychological. Collectively, then, these authors can be said to have engaged in unwarranted inferential leaps. By itself, brain research cannot be used to support particular instructional practices. It can, however, be used to support particular psychological theories of learning, which in turn can be used to design more effective forms of instruction.

FINAL THOUGHTS

Developmental psychologists, educational psychologists, and teachers tend to fall into one of four camps with respect to their orientation toward neuroscientific research (Byrnes & Fox, 1998): (1) those who readily accept (and sometimes overinterpret) the results of neuroscientific studies; (2) those who completely reject the neuroscientific approach and consider the results of neuroscientific studies to be meaningless; (3) those who are unfamiliar with, and indifferent toward, neuroscientific research; and (4) those who cautiously accept neuroscientific findings as being a provocative part of the total pattern of findings that have emerged from different corners of the cognitive and neural sciences. The present book was written to argue in favor of the fourth orientation. I hope that the readers of this book will likewise adopt the fourth orientation if they have not done so already. Moreover, I hope that educators and developmentalists will be motivated to conduct collaborative studies with their colleagues in the neurosciences in order to find answers to some of the fundamental questions I listed earlier. It is through these efforts that we will eventually learn whether a coherent integration of the psychological and neural sciences is truly possible.

Glossary

Afferent Stimulation: stimulation that runs along neural tracts away from the sensory and motor neurons in the hands, feet, and so on, to the brain. Pertains to the input fibers that bring sensory information to the brain.

Akinetic Mutism: a condition that sometimes follows brain injury to or lesions in the center, frontal region of the brain. The affected individual is disoriented, lethargic, and unable to speak.

Amygdala: a structure located on the lower, inner surface of the temporal lobe. It is thought to be important for emotional processing (especially for anger and fear).

Anencephalic: a condition of a fetus that involves having an underdeveloped brain (no cerebral hemispheres and only a rudimentary brainstem) and incomplete formation of the skull.

Angular Gyrus: a bulge in the cerebral cortex located near where the temporal lobe meets the parietal lobe (to find it, place your finger above and behind your ear).

Anterior (location term): the "face" portion or frontal surface of a structure when it is viewed laterally, that is, from the side (e.g., in the case of a head, the person's face is to the left and the back of the head is to the right). If a house were to be viewed from the side, the front door would be located on the anterior aspect; the back door would be located on the posterior aspect. An alternative term for anterior is *rostral* (the "nose" end of a four-legged animal viewed from the side).

Anterior Cingulate Gyrus: the frontal aspect of the cingulate gyrus, located in between the frontal lobes and the corpus callosum. Thought to be important for readiness for action; it is also active in nearly all cognitive tasks.

Arborization: the process of sprouting new dendrites on a neuron. It takes its name from the fact that the neuron looks like a tree that has sprouted new branches.

Areal Organization: the organization of areas in the cerebral cortex that have specific functions (e.g., the primary auditory areas in the temporal lobes vs. the primary visual areas in the occipital lobes).

Axon: the portion of a neuron that extends away from the cell body and nucleus and forms synapses with other neurons. Impulses (potentials) travel along the axon away from the cell body toward the next neuron in a series.

Broca's Area: a region of the left frontal lobe that is related to such things as the ability to speak, grammatical processing, word finding, and depression. It corresponds roughly to Brodmann Area 44.

Brodmann Areas: functional areas of the cortex assigned by a neuroanatomist named Brodmann. Until recently, the most commonly used system of brain reference to facilitate communication among scientists (e.g., in reference to questions such as "Where did the lesion occur?" or "Which areas of the cortex are active when people read words?").

Caudal (location term): the "tail" end of a structure (the opposite of the rostral or "nose" end). Generally synonymous with *posterior*. If a person's head were to be viewed from the side, the back of the head would be the caudal aspect of the head (the face would be the rostral aspect).

Cerebellum: a striated structure (with a braided appearance) located in the back of the head, behind the midbrain and below the posterior portion of the cerebral cortex. It is implicated in motor control, balance, and also some cognitive tasks.

Cerebral Cortex: the upper surface of the brain that has a bulbous or convoluted appearance. It is subdivided into various functional areas for vision, hearing, movement, speech, calculation, reasoning, and so on.

Cholinergic Tract: a tract of neurons that express the neurotransmitter acetylcholine into synapses. Neurons that cause muscles to contract are cholinergic.

Cingulate Gyrus: a gyrus, or extended bulge, running along the underside of the cerebral cortex. It extends from beneath the frontal lobes nearly to the occipital lobes, essentially covering the corpus callosum from front to back.

Computed Tomography (CT): a method for creating images of soft tissues like the brain. The apparatus makes 360-degree passes around a structure. An arc ring of detectors register the attenuated x-rays that have passed through the structure and compute a two-dimensional image from multiple passes.

Corpus Callosum: a bundle of fibers that connects regions of the two cerebral hemispheres together. Located beneath the cortex, it extends from anterior to posterior aspects of the brain.

Cortisol: one of the hormones secreted by the adrenal glands on top of the kidneys. It affects the level of glucose in the blood and is one of the hormones released under stressful situations. There are receptors for cortisol in the brain. Some scientists believe that it can promote cell death in the brain or retard the regeneration of neurons in the hippocampus.

Cytoarchitecture: the specific arrangement of neurons and glial cells in the brain (i.e., the fact that there are certain types of cells located in particular places and connected to each other in specific ways). Just as bricks and lumber make up the architecture of a house, brain cells make up the cytoarchitecture of the brain.

Dendrite: part of the neuron that branches away from the soma, or cell body. It has the capacity to receive impulses from other neurons. Synapses often form along its surface. When receptors in dendrites for neurotransmitters receive these neurotransmitters, an action potential begins (i.e., the neuron "fires").

Dopamine: one of the neurotransmitters in the brain.

Dopaminergic Neurons: neurons that express and have receptors for dopamine.

Dorsal (location term): the top or upper aspect of structures that have a top, bottom, front, and back. Synonymous with the term *superior*.

Dorsolateral Prefrontal Cortex (DFPC): a portion of the frontal lobes located near the top (hence, *dorso-*) and sides (hence, *lateral*) of these lobes in the two hemispheres. Thought to be important for higher forms of cognition such as working memory and inhibition.

Double Dissociation: a pair of experimental findings in which there is selective sparing of related cognitive functions. For example, imagine that damage to a region of the right parietal lobe produces a deficit in spatial working memory but leaves verbal working memory intact (Finding 1). Next, imagine that damage to a region of the left frontal lobe produces a deficit in verbal working memory but leaves spatial working memory intact (Finding 2). When both findings occur, we have a double dissociation.

Efferent Stimulation: stimulation that passes from the brain to sensory and motor neurons in the periphery (e.g., the hands or eyes).

Electroencephalogram (EEG): a recording of electrical activity in the brain. The output is a wave-like pattern that has negative components (valleys) and positive components (peaks) that occur across a second or so. Scientists try to link these peaks and valleys to specific cognitive events (e.g., detecting a target stimulus).

Epinephrine: a hormone secreted by the adrenal glands on top of the kidneys that increases sympathetic arousal (also known as adrenaline).

Executive Network: one of the three hypothesized attentional networks in the brain.

Experience-Dependent Plasticity: the ability of the nervous system to form new synaptic connections and reconfigure old connections in response to experience. Plasticity shows that the "wiring" of the brain (the pattern of connections) is dynamic, not constant over time.

Experience-Expectant Plasticity: the concept that some neural connections in the brain are set to form at, or slightly before, birth. All that is needed to "finish the wiring" is environmental stimulation that is typical for a given species.

Extrastriate Area: an area of the occipital lobe found just outside (hence, *extra-*) the striate area of this lobe. The striate area (the primary visual area) is so named for its striped appearance. Imagine concentric circles: the extrastriate area is like one of the outer rings and the striate area is like the innermost circle that surrounds the central sulcus.

Frontal Lobes: lobes of the cerebral cortex located in the anterior region of the brain (just beneath the forehead).

Functional Magnetic Resonance Imaging (fMRI): a kind of MRI that shows areas of the brain that are highly active during particular tasks. Relies on the assumption that blood flows to these active areas. Images are computed using the magnetic properties of substances in blood (e.g., water) and surrounding tissues.

Fusiform Gyrus: a gyrus located on the underside of the temporal lobe, near the front tip.

Gamma-Aminobutyric Acid (GABA): a neurotransmitter that is thought to have an inhibitory effect on postsynaptic cells.

Glial Cells: the other major kind of brain cells besides neurons. They probably do not participate in information processing but do play other roles such as structural support, myelin coatings, and neurotransmitter uptake.

Gyrus: any one of the elongated bulges that characterize the convoluted appearance of the cortex (plural is gyri).

Hippocampus: a region of the temporal lobes located on the inner, medial surface. Thought to be important to the formation or consolidation of new long-term memories.

Inferior (location term): the lower, bottom, or "underneath" aspect of a brain structure. If a ball on the floor had an inferior aspect, it would be the part that touches the floor.

Insula: the region of the brain that lies inside the fissure that separates the temporal and frontal lobes.

Laminar Organization: the organization of cortical cells into six horizontal layers, with different kinds of cells in each.

Lateral View: the view of a structure when looking at it from the side. The everyday term for the lateral view of a person's face is the *profile*.

Lesion: damage that occurs to a brain region due to a blow to the head, a stroke, and so on.

Locus Ceruleus (also Locus Coeruleus): a nucleus of the pons, located on the brainstem. The neurons of the locus ceruleus mostly use norepinephrine as neurotransmitter. It seems to play an important role in attention and arousal.

Magnetic Resonance Imaging (MRI): a technique for imaging slices of brain tissue and other internal organs. It relies on the magnetic properties of water and other substances.

Migration: during development, the process by which brain cells move from the proliferative zones in the neural tube to their proper location in the brain.

Myelination: the process by which the axons of larger neurons become covered with a fatty acid coating called *myelin*. Neurons with myelin conduct impulses 100 times faster than those without myelin.

Neocortex: literally, the "new bark of a tree." In the brain, it refers to the outer covering of the forebrain that is present in higher organisms. Also called the *cortex* for short, it consists of the frontal, parietal, temporal, and occipital lobes.

Neural Tube: a tube-like structure that appears in the embryonic phase of prenatal development (along the surface of the initially spherical embryo) and eventually gives rise to the brain and spinal cord.

Neuron: the other kind of brain cell besides glial cells. Patterns of neural activity are thought to correspond to thinking and information processing.

Neuronal Growth Factor: a substance that fosters the development of neurons (e.g., sprouting of new dendrites).

Neuroscience: the science concerned with the workings of the nervous system.

Neurulation: during brain development, the process by which the neural tube forms along the surface of the embryo.

Noradrenergic Neurons: neurons that express and respond to the neurotransmitter norepinephrine.

Norepinephrine: a hormone secreted by the adrenal glands that is also a neurotransmitter in the brain and spinal cord.

Occipital Lobe: the lobe of the cortex located in the back of the head (posterior aspect of the cortex). Areas of the occipital lobe are primarily involved in visual processing.

Orienting Network: one of the three hypothesized networks for controlling attention. Here, the network is responsible for shifting attention to a change in the environment.

Pallidum: also known as the *globus pallidus*. Together with the amygdala, the caudate nucleus, and the putamen, it comprises the subcortical ensemble known as the *basal ganglia*. It is located adjacent to the thalamus.

Parietal Lobe: one of the four lobes of the cortex located posterior to the frontal lobes but anterior and superior to the occipital lobes (lying approximately beneath a monk's baldspot). Thought to be important for spatial reasoning, math reasoning, and working memory.

Perisylvian Areas: areas of the cortex located near the Fissure of Sylvius that separates the frontal and parietal lobes from the temporal lobe. Broca's area and Wernicke's area are two of the perisylvian areas.

Phenylketonuria (PKU): children with PKU are unable to convert the amino acid phenylalanine into the amino acid tyrosine. As a result, they experience two main problems. First, high levels of phenylalanine in the bloodstream causes progressive brain damage and mental retardation. Second, tyrosine is a precursor to the neurotransmitter dopamine. Circuits comprised of dopaminergic neurons cannot work properly when the level of dopamine is too low.

Planum Temporale: a region of the cortex located near the junction of the temporal and parietal lobes (the posterior, superior surface of the superior temporal gyrus). Thought to be important for phonetic processing and linking sounds to printed words.

Plasticity: the ability of the nervous system to form new synaptic connections and reconfigure old connections in response to experience or injury. Plasticity shows that the "wiring" of the brain (the pattern of connections) is not constant over time but dynamic.

Positron Emission Tomography (PET): a method of brain imaging that assumes that blood is sent to areas of the brain that are especially active during a task. The instrument records the location of a radioactive isotope in the blood.

Posterior (location term): the back portion of a structure (to the right when one views the left side of a person's head). If a house were to be viewed from the left side, the anterior side would be the front-door side to the left; the posterior side would be the back-door side to the right.

Precuneus: a gyrus in the medial portion of the parietal lobe (also known as the superior parietal gyrus). It is bounded by the marginal sulcus and the parieto-occipital sulcus (which separates the parietal and occipital lobes).

Proliferation: the process of creating new brain cells during brain development.

Proliferative Zones: regions in the inner wall of the neural tube from which new brain cells emerge during brain development.

Pulvinar Nucleus: a nucleus located in the posterior portion of the thalamus.

Pyramidal Neurons: neurons whose cell bodies are shaped somewhat like pyramids. They comprise more than 80% of the neurons in the brain.

Raphe Nuclei: nuclei located in the medulla in the hindbrain (below the pons and the cerebellum).

Rostral (location term): synonymous with *anterior*. The "nose" or front end of an animal when viewed from the side (e.g., viewed from the left side, the head to the left, tail to the right). The nose on a person's face is rostral to the back of that person's head.

Serotonin: a neurotransmitter used by brain cells, especially those in the Raphe nuclei.

Splenium: the posterior, thickened portion of the corpus callosum.

Stellate Cells: star-shaped brain cells.

(Corpus) Striatum: one of the components of the basal ganglia located in front of, and lateral to, the thalamus in each cerebral hemisphere.

Subcortical Structures: various brain structures located underneath the cortex (e.g., the thalamus).

Substantia Nigra: a structure located near the basal ganglia that has a high concentration of dopamine. Its fibers input to a number of structures, including nuclei in the anterior portion of the thalamus.

Subtraction Technique: the experimental technique used to isolate brain areas responsible for a particular cognitive function. For example, the task of reading a word involves such things as visual fixation, attention, and recognition of a letter pattern. To isolate the areas specifically responsible for letter recognition, one has to get activations for tasks that require *only* visual fixation and *only* attention. Then one subtracts the activations for fixation and attention away from the activation for letter recognition to determine the areas that are specifically active for letter recognition.

Sulcus: a groove in the cortex.

Superior (location term): synonymous with *dorsal*. The upper aspect (or top surface) of a structure.

Superior Colliculus: a subcortical structure located just below the thalamus. Thought to be important for controlling eye movements and shifting attention.

Superior Temporal Sulcus: a groove that runs along the top surface of the temporal lobe.

Synaptic Density: the number of synapses per unit area (e.g., 1,000 synapses per micron).

Synaptogenesis: the process of forming new, stable synapses between neurons.

Tegmental Area: an area of the pons and some adjacent portions of the brainstem.

Temporal Lobe: one of the four lobes of the brain that lie beneath the temples. The temporal lobes are inferior to the frontal and parietal lobes, and anterior to the occipital lobes. They are involved in auditory processing (both hemispheres) and certain language skills (left hemispheres in most right-handed people and vice versa).

Teratogen: any foreign substance that causes abnormalities in a developing embryo or fetus.

Thalamus: a subcortical structure that sends afferent projections to specific areas of the cortex. Said to be a "relay" station for afferent input.

Thymus: a gland located in the upper chest under the breastbone in humans. Beginning in fetal life, it plays an important role in the development of the body's immune system. The thymus produces white blood cells known as *lymphocytes*, which kill foreign cells and stimulate other immune cells to produce antibodies. The gland grows throughout childhood until puberty and then gradually decreases in size.

Transcranial Magnetic Stimulation: a noninvasive technique for localizing the function of cortical areas that involves sending a magnetic pulse through the skull to brain tissue underneath. Said to cause temporary "virtual lesions."

Vagal Tone: neural control of the heart via the vagus nerve. Monitored as an index of homeostasis.

Ventral (location term): synonymous with *inferior*. Refers to the bottom or lower aspect of a structure.

Vigilance Network: one of three hypothesized attentional networks. The vigilance network is operative when a person is waiting for the occurrence of some event.

Wernicke's Aphasia: a language disorder in which an individual can engage in fluent but incoherent speech. In addition, the individual cannot comprehend things said to him or her. This disorder has been found mainly when damage occurs in the left hemisphere in Brodmann Areas 22 and 39 (superior, posterior temporal lobe and the angular gyrus).

Yerkes–Dodson Law: a scientific law based on the observation that animals (including humans) seem to learn more when they are in a state of moderate arousal than when they are in state of either low arousal or high arousal (which can be charted as an inverted-U-shaped learning curve).

References

Adams, M. J. (1990). *Beginning to read.* Cambridge, MA: Harvard University Press.

Alba, J. W., & Hasher, L. (1982). Is memory schematic? *Psychological Bulletin, 93,* 203–231.

Alexander, J. E., O'Boyle, M. W., & Benbow, C. P. (1996). Developmentally advanced EEG alpha power in gifted male and female adolescents. *International Journal of Psychophysiology, 23,* 25–31.

American Psychiatric Association. (1994). *Diagnostic and statistical manual of mental disorders* (4th ed.). Washington, DC: Author.

Anderson, J. R. (1990). *Cognitive psychology and its implications* (3rd ed.). New York: Freeman.

Anderson, J. R. (1993). Problem solving and learning. *American Psychologist, 48,* 35–44.

Anderson, J. R. (1995). *Learning and memory: An integrated approach.* New York: Wiley.

Anderson, J. R., & Schooler, L. J. (1991). Reflections on the environment in memory. *Psychological Science, 2,* 396–408.

Applegate, B., Lahey, B.B., Hart, E. L., Biederman, J., Hynd, G. W., Barkley, R. A., Ollendick, T., Frick, P. J., Greenhill, L., McBurnett, K., Newcorn, J. H., Kerdyk, L., Garfinkel, B., Waldman, I., & Shaffer, D. (1997). Validity of the age-of-onset criterion for ADHD: A report from the DSM-IV field trials. *Journal of the American Academy of Child and Adolescent Psychiatry, 36,* 1211–1221.

Aston-Jones, G., Rajkowski, J., & Cohen, J. (1999). Role of locus coeruleus in attention and behavioral flexibility. *Biological Psychiatry, 46,* 1309–1320.

Atkinson, R. C., & Shiffrin, R. M. (1968). Human memory: A proposed system and its control processes. In K. W. Spence & J. T. Spence (Eds.), *The psychology of learning and motivation: Advances in research and theory* (Vol. 2, pp. 89–195). New York: Academic Press.

Baddeley, A. (1999). *Essentials of human memory.* Philadelphia: Psychology Press.

Barch, D. M., Braver, T. S., Nystrom, L. E., Forman, S. D., Noll, D. C., & Cohen, J. D. (1997). Dissociating working memory from task difficulty in human prefrontal cortex. *Neuropsychologia, 35,* 1373–1380.

Barkley, R. A. (1997). Behavioral inhibition, sustained attention, and executive functions: Constructing a unifying theory of ADHD. *Psychological Review, 121,* 65–94.

Barkley, R. A., & Bierderman, J. (1997). Toward a broader definition of the age-of-onset criterion for attention-deficit hyperactivity disorder. *Journal of the American Academy of Child and Adolescent Psychiatry, 36,* 1204–1210.

Barr, H. M., & Streissguth, A. P. (1991). Caffeine use during pregnancy and child outcome: A 7-year prospective study. *Neurotoxicology and Teratology, 13*, 441–448.

Barr, H. M., Streissguth, A. P., Darby, B. L., & Sampson, P. D. (1990). Prenatal exposure to alcohol, caffeine, tobacco, and aspirin: Effects on fine and gross motor performance in 4-year-old children. *Developmental Psychology, 26*, 339–348.

Beaton, A. (1997). The relation of planum temporale asymmetry and morphology of the corpus callosum to handedness, gender, and dyslexia: A review of the evidence. *Brain and Language, 60*, 255–322.

Begley, S. (1996, February). Your child's brain. *Newsweek*, pp. 55–62.

Bellinger, D., & Needleman, H. L. (1994). Developmental toxicity of methyl mercury. In H. L. Needleman & D. Bellinger (Eds.), *Prenatal exposure to toxicants: Developmental consequences* (pp. 89–111). Baltimore: Johns Hopkins University Press.

Benbow, C. P. (1986). Physiological correlates of extreme intellectual precocity. *Neuropsychologia, 24*, 719–725.

Benbow, C. P. (1988). Sex differences in mathematical reasoning ability in intellectually talented preadolescents: Their nature, effects, and possible causes. *Behavioral and Brain Sciences, 11*, 169–232.

Benton, S. L., Glover, J. A., Monkowski, P.G., & Shaughnessy, M. (1983). Decision difficulty and recall of prose. *Journal of Educational Psychology, 75*, 727–742.

Bernstein, P. L. (1996). *Against the gods: The remarkable story of risk.* New York: Wiley.

Block, N. (1990). The computer model of the mind. In D. N. Osherson & E. E. Smith (Eds.), *Thinking* (pp. 245–289). Cambridge, MA: MIT Press.

Bransford, J. D., Brown, A. L., & Cocking, R. R. (1999). *How people learn: Brain, mind, experience, and school.* Washington, DC: National Academy Press.

Breedlove, S. M. (1994). Sexual differentiation of the human nervous system. *Annual Review of Psychology, 45*, 389–418.

Bremner, J. D. (1999). Does stress damage the brain? *Biological Psychiatry, 45*, 797–805.

Broadbent, D. E. (1958). *Perception and communication.* London: Pergamon Press.

Bruer, J. T. (1997). Education and the brain: A bridge too far. *Educational Researcher, 26*, 4–16.

Bruer, J. T. (1998). Brain science, brain fiction. *Educational Leadership, 56*, 14–18.

Bruner, J. S. (1966). *Toward a theory of instruction.* Cambridge, MA: Belknap Press of Harvard University Press.

Bryant, P. E., MacLean, M., Bradley, L., & Crossland, J. (1990). Rhyme and alliteration, phoneme detection, and learning to read. *Developmental Psychology, 26*, 429–438.

Bryden, M. P., McManus, I. C., & Bulman-Fleming, M. B. (1994). Evaluating the empirical support for the Geschwind–Behan–Galaburda model of cerebral lateralization. *Brain and Cognition, 26*, 103–167.

Bullock, M., Gelman, R., & Baillargeon, R. (1982). The development of causal reasoning. In W. J. Friedman (Ed.), *The developmental psychology of time* (pp. 209–254). New York: Academic Press.

Byrnes, J. P. (1992). The conceptual basis of procedural learning. *Cognitive Development, 7*, 235–257.

Byrnes, J. P. (1999). The nature and development of representation: Forging a synthesis of competing approaches. In I. Sigel (Ed.), *Development of representation* (pp. 273–294). Mahwah, NJ: Erlbaum.

Byrnes, J. P. (2001). *Cognitive development and learning in instructional contexts.* Needham Heights, MA: Allyn & Bacon.

Byrnes, J. P., & Fox, N. A. (1998). The educational relevance of research in cognitive neuroscience. *Educational Psychology Review, 10*, 297–342.

Byrnes, J. P., & Takahira, S. (1994). Why some students perform well and others perform poorly on SAT-math items. *Contemporary Educational Psychology, 19*, 63–78.

Cahill, L., & McGaugh, J. L. (1998). Modulation of memory storage. In L. R. Squire & S. M. Kosslyn (Eds.), *Findings and current opinion in cognitive neuroscience* (pp. 85–90). Cambridge, MA: MIT Press.

Caine, G., & Caine, R. N. (1997). *Education on the edge of possibility.* Alexandria, VA: Association for Supervision and Curriculum Development.

Camras, L. A. (1994). Two aspects of emotional development: Expression and elicitation. In P. Ekman & R. J. Davidson (Eds.), *The nature of emotion* (pp. 347–351). New York: Oxford University Press.

Canli, T., Desmond, J. E., Zhao, Z., Glover, G., & Gabrieli, J. D. E. (1998). Hemispheric asymmetry for emotional stimuli detected with fMRI. *Neuroreport, 9*, 3233–3239.

Case, R., & Okamoto, Y. (1996). The role of central conceptual structures in the development of children's thought. *Monographs of the Society for Research in Child Development, 61*, v–265.

Casey, B. J., Cohen, J. D., Noll, D. C., Schneider, W., Giedd, J. N., & Rappaport, J. L. (1996). Functional magnetic resonance imaging: Studies of cognition. In E. D. Bigler (Ed.), *Neuroimaging: Vol. 2. Clinical applications* (pp. 299–330). New York: Plenum Press.

Chenn, A., Braisted, J. E., McConnell, S. K., & O'Leary, D. D. M. (1997). Development of the cerebral cortex: Mechanisms controlling cell fate, laminar and areal patterning, and axonal connectivity. In W. M. Cowan, T. M. Jessell, & S. L. Zipursky (Eds.), *Molecular and cellular approaches to neural development* (pp. 440–473). New York: Oxford University Press.

Cherry, S. R., & Phelps, M. E. (1996). Imaging brain function with positron emission tomography. In A. W. Toga & J. C. Mazziotta (Eds.), *Brain mapping: The methods* (pp. 191–219). Orlando, FL: Academic Press.

Clore, G. L. (1994). Why emotions require cognition. In P. Ekman & R. J. Davidson (Eds.), *The nature of emotion* (pp. 181–191). New York: Oxford University Press.

Cohen, M. S. (1996). Rapid MRI and functional applications. In A. W. Toga & J. C. Mazziotta (Eds.), *Brain mapping: The methods* (pp. 191–219). Orlando, FL: Academic Press.

Coyle, J. T., Oster-Granite, M. L., Reeves, R. H., & Gearhart, J. D. (1988). Down syndrome, Alzheimer's disease, and the trisomy 16 mouse. *Trends in the Neurosciences, 11*, 390–394.

Craik, F. I. M., & Lockhart, R. S. (1972). Levels of processing: A framework for memory research. *Journal of Verbal Learning and Verbal Behavior, 11*, 671–684.

Csikszentmihalyi, M. (1998). *Finding flow: The psychology of engagement with everyday life.* New York: Basic Books.

Davidson, R. J. (1992). Emotion and affective style. *Psychological Science, 3*, 39–43.

Davidson, R. J., & Ekman, P. (1994). Afterword. In P. Ekman & R. J. Davidson (Eds.), *The nature of emotion* (pp. 261–262). New York: Oxford University Press.

DeFries, J. C., Gillis, J. J., & Wadsworth, S. J. (1993). Genes and genders: A twin study of reading disability. In A. M. Galaburda (Ed.), *Dyslexia and development: Neurobiological development of extraordinary brains* (pp. 187–204). Cambridge, MA: Harvard University Press.

Dehaene, S. (1996). The organization of brain activations in number comparison: Event-related potentials and the additive factors method. *Journal of Cognitive Neuroscience, 8*, 47–68.

Dehaene, S., & Cohen, L. (1997). Cerebral pathways for calculation: Double dissociation between rote verbal and quantitative knowledge of arithmetic. *Cortex, 33*, 219–250.

Dehaene, S., Tzourio, N., Frak, V., Raynaud, L., Cohen, L., Mehler, J., & Mazoyer, B. (1996). Cerebral activations during number multiplication and comparison: A PET study. *Neuropsychologia, 34,* 1097–1106.

Diamond, A., Prevor, M. B., Callender, G., & Druin, D. P. (1997). Prefrontal cortex cognitive deficits in children treated early and continuously for PKU. *Monographs of the Society for Research in Child Development, 62* (Serial No. 252, pp. 1–205).

Dix, T., Ruble, D. N., Grusec, J. E., & Nixon, S. (1986). Social cognition in parents: Inferential and affective reactions to children of three age levels. *Child Development, 57,* 879–894.

Dodge, D. T., & Heronman, C. (1999). *Building your baby's brain: A parent's guide to the first five years.* Washington, DC: Teaching Strategies.

Drevets, W. C., & Raichle, M. E. (1995). Positron emission tomographic imaging studies of human emotional disorders. In M. S. Gazzaniga (Ed.), *The cognitive neurosciences* (pp. 1153–1164). Cambridge, MA: MIT Press.

Driesen, N. R., & Raz, N. (1995). The influence of sex, age, and handedness on corpus callosum morphology: A meta-analysis. *Psychobiology, 23,* 240–247.

Dunn, J. (1994). Experience and understanding of emotions, relationships, and membership in a particular culture. In P. Ekman & R. J. Davidson (Eds.), *The nature of emotion* (pp. 353–355). New York: Oxford University Press.

Edelman, G. R. (1992). *Bright air, brilliant fire: On the matter of the mind.* New York: Basic Books.

Ekman, P. (1994). All emotions are basic. In P. Ekman, & R. J. Davidson (Eds.), *The nature of emotion* (pp. 15–19). New York: Oxford University Press.

Ekman, P., & Davidson, R. J. (Eds.). (1994). *The nature of emotion.* New York: Oxford University Press.

Elbert, T., Pantev, C., Wienbruch, C., Rockstroh, B., & Taub, E. (1995). Increased cortical representation of the fingers of the left hand in string players. *Science, 270,* 305–307.

Engel, S. A., Rumelhart, D. E., Wandell, B. A., Lee, A. T., Glover, G. H., Chichilnisky, E. J., & Shaden, M. N. (1994). fMRI of human visual cortex. *Nature, 369,* 525–526.

Ericsson, K. A. (1996). *The road to excellence: The acquisition of expert performance in the arts and science, sports, and games.* Mahwah, NJ: Erlbaum.

Feitelson, D., Tehori, B. Z., & Levinberg-Green, D. (1982). How effective is early instruction in reading? Experimental evidence. *Merrill–Palmer Quarterly, 28,* 485–494.

Finlay, B. L., & Darlington, R. B. (1995). Linked regularities in the development and evolution of mammalian brains. *Science, 268,* 1578–1584.

Fisher, H., Wik, G., & Fredrikson, M. (1996). Functional neuroanatomy of robbery reexperience. Affective memories studied with PET. *Neuroreport, 7,* 2081–2086.

Flavell, J. H., Miller, P. H., & Miller, S. A. (1993). *Cognitive development* (3rd ed.). Englewood Cliffs, NJ: Prentice-Hall.

Folstein, S. E. (1989). *Huntington's disease: A disorder of families.* Baltimore: Johns Hopkins University Press.

Fowler, W. (1971). A developmental learning strategy for early reading in a laboratory nursery school. *Interchange, 2,* 106–124.

Fox, N. A. (1991). If it's not left, it's right: Electroencephalograph asymmetry and the development of emotion. *American Psychologist, 46,* 863–872.

Fox, N. A., & Bell, M. A. (1990). Electrophysiological indices of frontal lobe development: Relations to cognitive and affective behavior in human infants over the first year of life. In A. Diamond (Ed.), *The development and neural bases of higher cortical functions* (pp. 677–704). New York: New York Academy of Sciences.

Frijda, N. (1994). Emotions are functional, most of the time. In P. Ekman & R. J. Davidson (Eds.), *The nature of emotion* (pp. 112–122). New York: Oxford University Press.

Galaburda, A. M. (1993). *Dyslexia and development: Neurobiological aspects of extra-ordinary brains*. Cambridge, MA: Harvard University Press.

Garber, J., & Dodge, K. A. (1991). *The development of emotion regulation and dysregulation*. New York: Cambridge University Press.

Garner, R. (1987). Strategies for reading and studying expository texts. *Educational Psychologist, 22*, 299–312.

Garrett, M. F. (1990). Sentence processing. In D. N. Osherson & H. Lasnik (Eds.), *An invitation to cognitive science: Vol. 1. Language* (pp. 133–175). Cambridge, MA: MIT Press.

Gayan, J., Smith, S. D., Cherny, S. S., Cardon, L. R., Fulker, D. W., Brower, A. M., Olson, R. K., Pennington, B. F., & DeFries, J. C. (1999). Quantitative-trait locus for specific language and reading deficits. *American Journal of Human Genetics, 64*, 157–164.

Geary, D.C. (1993). Mathematical disabilities: Cognitive, neuropsychological, and genetic components. *Psychological Bulletin, 114*, 345–362.

Geary, D. C. (1998). What is the function of mind and brain? *Educational Psychology Review, 10*, 377–388.

Geschwind, N., & Behan, P. (1982). Left-handedness: Association with immune disease, migraine, and developmental learning disorder. *Proceedings of the National Academy of Sciences, 79*, 5097–5100.

Geschwind, N., & Galaburda, A. M. (1985). Cerebral lateralization: Biological mechanisms, associations, and pathology, 1: A hypothesis and a program for research. *Archives of Neurology, 42*, 428–459.

Geschwind, N., & Galaburda, A. M. (1987). *Cerebral lateralization*. Cambridge, MA: MIT Press.

Gevins, A. (1996). Electrophysiological imaging of brain function. In A. W. Toga & J. C. Mazziotta (Eds.), *Brain mapping: The methods* (pp. 259–274). Orlando, FL: Academic Press.

Gick, M. L., & Holyoak, K. J. (1983). Schema induction and analogical transfer. *Cognitive Psychology, 15*, 1–38.

Giedd, J. N., Rumsey, J. M., Castellanos, F. X., Rajapakse, J. C., Kaysen, D., Vaituzis, A. C., Vauss, Y. C., Hamburger, S. D., & Rapoport, J. L. (1996). A quantitative MRI study of the corpus callosum in children and adolescents. *Developmental Brain Research, 91*, 274–280.

Glover, J. A., Ronning, R. R., & Bruning, R. H. (1990). *Cognitive psychology for teachers*. New York: Macmillan.

Goldman-Rakic, P. S. (1986). Setting the stage: Neural development before birth. In S. L. Peterson, K. A. Klivington, & R. W. Peterson (Eds.), *The brain, cognition, and education* (pp. 233–258). New York: Academic Press.

Goldman-Rakic, P. S. (1992). Working memory and the mind. *Scientific American, 90*, 111–117.

Goldman-Rakic, P. S. (1994). Specification of higher cortical functions. In S. H. Broman & J. Grafman (Eds.), *Atypical cognitive deficits in developmental disorders: Implications for brain function* (pp. 3–18). Mahwah, NJ: Erlbaum.

Goldstein, D. M. (1978). Cognitive–linguistic functioning and learning to read in preschoolers. *Journal of Educational Psychology, 68*, 680–688.

Goodman, C. S., & Tessier-Lavigne, M. (1997). Molecular mechanisms of axon guidance and target recognition. In W. M. Cowan, T. M. Jessell, & S. L. Zipursky (Eds.), *Molecular and cellular approaches to neural development* (pp. 108–137). New York: Oxford University Press.

Graesser, A., Golding, J. M. & Long, D. L. (1991). Narrative representation and comprehension. In R. Barr, M. L. Kamil, P. Mosenthal, & P. D. Pearson (Eds.), *Handbook of reading research* (Vol 2, pp. 171–205). New York: Longman.

Greenough, W. T., Black, J. E., & Wallace, C. S. (1987). Experience and brain development. *Child Development, 58,* 539–559.

Gunnar, M. R., & Barr, R. G. (1998). Stress, early brain development, and behavior. *Infants and Young Children, 11,* 1–14.

Halgren, E., & Marinkovic, K. (1995). Neurophysiological networks integrating human emotions. In M. S. Gazzaniga (Ed.), *The cognitive neurosciences* (pp. 1137–1151). Cambridge, MA: MIT Press.

Halpern, D. F. (1992). *Sex differences in cognitive abilities* (2nd ed.). Hillsdale, NJ: Erlbaum.

Hassold, T., Sherman, S., & Hunt, P. A. (1995). The origin of trisomy in humans. In C. J. Epstein, T. Hassold, I. T. Lott, L. Nadel, & D. Patterson (Eds.), *Etiology and pathogenesis of Down syndrome* (pp. 1–12). New York: Wiley-Liss.

Hiebert, J., & LeFevre, P. (1987). Conceptual and procedural knowledge in mathematics: An introductory analysis. In J. Hiebert (Ed.), *Conceptual and procedural knowledge in mathematics* (pp. 1–27). Hillsdale, NJ: Erlbaum.

Hillyard, S. A., Mangun, G. R., Woldorff, M. G., & Luck, S. J. (1995). Neural systems mediating selective attention. In M. S. Gazzaniga (Ed.), *The cognitive neurosciences* (pp. 665–681). Cambridge, MA: MIT Press.

Hinds, T. S., West, W. L., Knight, E. M., & Harland, B. F. (1996). The effect of caffeine on pregnancy outcome variables. *Nutrition Review, 54,* 203–207.

Hintzman, D. L. (1986). "Schema abstraction" in a multiple-trace memory model. *Psychological Review, 93,* 411–428.

Hittmair-Delazer, M., Semenza, C., & Denes, G. (1994). Concepts and facts in calculation. *Brain, 117,* 715–728.

Hubel, D. H., & Wiesel, T. N. (1962). Receptive fields, binocular interaction, and functional architecture in the cat's visual cortex. *Journal of Physiology, 160,* 106–154.

Huttenlocher, P. R. (1993). Morphometric study of human cerebral cortex development. In M. H. Johnson (Ed.), *Brain development and cognition: A reader* (pp. 112–124). Cambridge, MA: Blackwell.

Hynd, G. W., Marshall, R., & Gonzales, J. (1991). Learning disabilities and presumed central nervous system dysfunction. *Learning Disability Quarterly, 14,* 283–296.

Iran-Nejad, A., Hidi, S., & Wittrock, M. C. (1992). Reconceptualizing relevance in education from a biological perspective. *Educational Psychologist, 27,* 407–414.

Izard, C. E. (1994). Intersystem connections. In P. Ekman, & R. J. Davidson (Eds.), *The nature of emotion* (pp. 356–361). New York: Oxford University Press.

Izard, C. E., Fantauzzo, C. A., Castle, J. M., Haynes, O. M., Rayias, M. F., & Putnam, P. H. (1995). The ontogeny and significance of infant's facial expressions in the first nine months of life. *Developmental Psychology, 31,* 997–1013.

Jackson, N. E. (1992). Precocious reading ability: Origins, structure, and predictive significance. In P. S. Klein & A. J. Tannenbaum (Eds.), *To be young and gifted* (pp. 171–203). Norwood, NJ: Ablex.

James, W. (1890). *The principles of psychology.* New York: Holt.

Jensen, E. (1998). *Teaching with the brain in mind.* Alexandria, VA: Association for Supervision and Curriculum Development.

Johnson, M. H. (1993). *Brain development and cognition: A reader.* Cambridge, MA: Blackwell.

Johnson, M. H. (1997). *Developmental cognitive neuroscience: An introduction.* Cambridge, MA: Blackwell.

Just, M. A., & Carpenter, P. A. (1987). *The psychology of reading and language comprehension*. Boston: Allyn & Bacon.

Kandel, E. R. (1991). Nerve cells and behavior. In E. R. Kandel, J. H. Schwartz, & T. M. Jessell (Eds.), *Principles of neural science* (3rd ed., pp. 18–32). Norwalk, CT: Appleton & Lange.

Kelley, D. B. (1993). Androgens and brain development: Possible contributions to developmental dyslexia. In A. M. Galaburda (Ed.), *Dyslexia and development: Neurobiological aspects of extra-ordinary brains* (pp. 21–41). Cambridge, MA: Harvard University Press.

Kemper, T. L. (1988). Neuropathology of Down Syndrome. In L. Nadel (Ed.), *The psychobiology of Down syndrome* (pp. 269–289). Cambridge, MA: MIT Press.

Killcross, S., Robbins, T. W., & Everitt, B. J. (1997). Different types of fear-conditioned behaviour mediated by separate nuclei within amygdala. *Nature, 388,* 377–380.

Kintsch, W. (1974). *The representation of meaning in memory*. Hillsdale, NJ: Erlbaum.

Kintsch, W. (1982). Text representations. In W. Otto & S. White (Eds.), *Reading expository material* (pp. 87–102). New York: Academic Press.

Kleim, J. A., Swain, R. A., Armstrong, K. A., Napper, R. M. A., Jones, T. A., & Greenough, W. T. (1998). Selective synaptic plasticity within the cerebellar cortex following complex motor skill learning. *Neurobiology of Learning and Memory, 69,* 274–289.

Knopik, V. S., Alarcon, M., & DeFries, J. C. (1997). Common and specific gender influences on individual differences in reading performance: A twin study. *Personality and Individual Differences, 25,* 269–277.

Kosslyn, S. M., & Intriligator, J. M. (1992). Is cognitive neuropsychology plausible?: The perils of sitting on a one-legged stool. *Journal of Cognitive Neuroscience, 4,* 96–106.

Kosslyn, S. M., & Koenig, O. (1992). *Wet mind: The new cognitive neuroscience*. New York: Free Press.

Kuhl, P. K. (1998). Learning and representation in speech and language. In L. R. Squire & S. M. Kosslyn (Eds.), *Findings and current opinion in cognitive neuroscience* (pp. 353–364). Cambridge, MA: MIT Press.

Kutas, M., & Van Petten, C. (1988). Event-related brain potential studies of language. In P. Ackles, J. R. Jennings, & M. Coles (Eds.), *Advances in psychophysiology* (pp. 139–153). Greenwich, CT: JAI Press.

Lane, R. D., Reiman, E. M., Ahern, G. L., Schwartz, G. E., & Davidson, R. J. (1997). Neuroanatomical correlates of happiness, sadness, and disgust. *American Journal of Psychiatry, 154,* 926–933.

Lasnick, H. (1990). Syntax. In D. N. Osherson & H. Lasnik (Eds.), *An invitation to cognitive science: Vol. 1. Language* (pp. 5–22). Cambridge, MA: MIT Press.

Lazarus, R. S. (1991). *Emotion and adaptation*. New York: Oxford University Press.

Lazarus, R. S. (1994). Meaning and emotional development. In P. Ekman, & R. J. Davidson (Eds.), *The nature of emotion* (pp. 362–366). New York: Oxford University Press.

LeDoux, J. E. (1995). In search of an emotional system in the brain: Leaping from fear to emotion and consciousness. In M. S. Gazzaniga (Ed.), *The cognitive neurosciences* (pp. 1049–1061). Cambridge, MA: MIT Press.

Lindsley, D. B., & Wicke, J. D. (1974). The EEG: Autonomous electrical activity in man and animals. In R. Thompson & M. N. Patterson (Eds.), *Bioelectrical recording techniques* (pp. 3–83). New York: Academic Press.

Lowery, L. (1998). How new science curriculums reflect brain research. *Educational Leadership, 56,* 27–30.

Luria, A. R. (1973). *The working brain*. New York: Basic Books.

Markman, E. M. (1981). Comprehension monitoring. In W. P. Dickson (Ed.), *Children's oral communication skills* (pp. 61–84). New York: Academic Press.

Markovits, Z., & Sowder, J. (1994). Developing number sense: An intervention study in grade 7. *Journal for Research in Mathematics Education, 25*, 4–29.

Marr, D. (1982). *Vision: A computational investigation into the human representation and processing of visual information.* San Francisco: Freeman.

Martin, A., Haxby, J. V., Lalonde, F. M., Wiggs, C. L., & Ungerleider, L. G. (1995, October). Discrete cortical regions associated with knowledge of color and knowledge of action. *Science, 270,* 102–105.

Martin, A., Wiggs, C. L., Ungerleider, L. G., & Haxby, J. V. (1996). Neural correlates of category-specific knowledge. *Nature, 379,* 649–652.

Masten, A. S., & Coatsworth, J. D. (1998). The development of competence in favorable and unfavorable environments. *American Psychologist, 53,* 205–220.

Mayer, R. E. (1982). Memory for algebra story problems. *Journal of Educational Psychology, 74,* 199–216.

McCarthy, R. A., & Warrington, E. K. (1990). *Cognitive neuropsychology: A clinical introduction.* San Diego, CA: Academic Press.

McCloskey, M., Aliminosa, D., & Sokol, S. M. (1991). Facts, rules, and procedures in normal calculation: Evidence from multiple single-patient studies of impaired arithmetic fact retrieval. *Brain and Cognition, 17,* 154–203.

McCloskey, M., Caramazza, A., & Basili, A. (1985). Cognitive mechanisms in number processing and calculation: Evidence from dyscalculia. *Brain and Cognition, 4,* 171–196.

McDaniel, M. A., Einstein, G. O., Dunay, P. K., & Cobb, R. S. (1986). Encoding difficulty and memory: Toward a unifying theory. *Journal of Memory and Language, 25,* 645–656.

McDaniel, M. A., Waddell, P. J., & Einstein, G. O. (1988). A contextual account of the generation effect: A three factor theory. *Journal of Memory and Language, 27,* 521–536.

McEwen, B. S. (1995). Stressful experience, brain, and emotions: Developmental, genetic, and hormonal influences. In M. S. Gazzaniga (Ed.), *The cognitive neurosciences* (pp. 1117–1135). Cambridge MA: MIT Press.

Metsala, J. L. (1999). Young children's phonological awareness and nonword repetition as a function of vocabulary development. *Journal of Educational Psychology, 91,* 3–19.

Meyer, B. J. F. (1985). Prose analysis: Purposes, procedures, and problems. In B. K. Britton & J. B. Black (Eds.), *Understanding expository text* (pp. 11–66). Hillsdale, NJ: Erlbaum.

Mishkin, M., & Murray, E. A. (1998). Stimulus recognition. In L. R. Squire & S. M. Kosslyn (Eds.), *Findings and current opinion in cognitive neuroscience* (pp. 67–74). Cambridge, MA: MIT Press.

Moonen, C. T. W. (1995). Imaging of human brain activation with functional MRI. *Biological Psychiatry, 37,* 141–143.

Morphett, M., & Washburn, C. (1931). When should children begin to read? *Elementary School Journal, 31,* 496–503.

Morris, J. S., Frith, C. D., Perrett, D. I., Rowland, D., Young, A. W., Calder, A. J., & Dolan, R. J. (1996). A differential neural response in the human amygdala for fearful and happy facial expressions. *Nature, 383,* 812–815.

Moyer, K. E. (1980). *Neuroanatomy.* New York: Harper & Row.

Nathanielsz, P. W. (1999). *Life in the womb: The origin of health and disease.* New York: Prometheon Press.

National Council of Teachers of Mathematics. (1998). *Principles and standards for school mathematics: Discussion draft.* Reston, VA: Author.

Neisser, U. (1967). *Cognitive psychology.* New York: Appleton-Century-Crofts.

Newell, A., & Rosenbloom, P.S. (1981). Mechanisms of skills acquisition and the law of practice. In J. R. Anderson (Ed.), *Cognitive skills and their acquisition* (pp. 1–55). Hillsdale, NJ: Erlbaum.

Newell, A., & Simon, H. A. (1972). *Human problem solving*. Englewood Cliffs, NJ: Prentice-Hall.

O'Boyle, M. W., & Benbow, C. P. (1990). Enhanced right hemisphere involvement during cognitive processing may relate to intellectual precocity. *Neuropsychologia, 28,* 211–216.

O'Boyle, M. W., & Gill, H. S. (1998). On the relevance of research findings in cognitive neuroscience to educational practice. *Educational Psychology Review, 10,* 397–410.

Oldfield, R. C. (1971). The assessment and analysis of handedness: Edinburgh inventory. *Neuropsychologia, 9,* 97–113.

Paivio, A. (1971). *Imagery and verbal processes*. New York: Holt, Rinehart & Winston.

Paris, S. G., Wasik, B. A., & Turner, J. C. (1991). The development of strategic readers. In R. Barr, M. L. Kamil, P. B. Mosenthal, & P. D. Pearson (Eds.), *Handbook of reading research* (Vol. 2, pp. 609–640). New York: Longman.

Pesenti, M., Seron, X., & Van Der Linden, M. (1994). Selective impairment as evidence for mental organization of arithmetical facts: BB, a case of preserved subtraction? *Cortex, 30,* 661–671.

Petersen, S. E., Fox, P. T., Snyder, A. Z., & Raichle, M. E. (1990). Activation of extrastriate and frontal cortical areas by visual words and word-like stimuli. *Science, 240,* 1041–1044.

Peterson, P. L., Fennema, E., Carpenter, T. P., & Loef, M. (1989). Teacher's pedagogical content beliefs in mathematics. *Cognition and Instruction, 6,* 1–40.

Pinker, S. (1997). *How the mind works*. New York: Norton.

Pintrich, P. R., & Schunk, D. H. (1996). *Motivation in education: Theory, research, and applications*. Englewood Cliffs, NJ: Merrill.

Plude, D. J., Enns, J. T., & Brodeur, D. (1994). The development of selective attention: A life-span view. *Acta Psychologica, 86,* 227–272.

Pollitt, E., Gorman, K. S., Engle, P. L., Martorell, R., & Rivera, J. (1993). Early supplemental feeding and cognition: Effects over two decades. *Monographs of the Society for Research in Child Development, 58*(Serial No. 235, pp. v–99).

Porges, S. W. (1995). Orienting in a defensive world: Mammalian modification of our evolutionary heritage. A polyvagal theory. *Psychophysiology, 32,* 301–318.

Posner, M. I. (1995). Attention in cognitive neuroscience: An overview. In M. S. Gazzaniga (Ed.), *The cognitive neurosciences* (pp. 615–624). Cambridge MA: MIT Press.

Posner, M. I. (1997, April). *Cognitive neuroscience and the development of attention*. Address delivered at the biennial meeting of the Society for Research in Child Development, Washington, DC.

Posner, M. I., Peterson, S. E., Fox, P. T., & Raichle, M. E. (1988). Localization of cognitive operations in the human brain. *Science, 240,* 1627–1631.

Posner, M. I., & Raichle, M. E. (1994). *Images of mind*. New York: Scientific American Library.

Pressley, M. (1997). The cognitive science of reading: Comments. *Contemporary Educational Psychology, 22,* 247–259.

Pressley, M., Almasi, J., Schuder, T., Bergman, J., Hite, S., El-Dinary, P. B., & Brown, R. (1994). Transactional instruction of comprehension strategies: The Montgomery County Maryland SAIL program. *Reading and Writing Quarterly, 10,* 5–19.

Pressley, M., Levin, J., & Delaney, H. D. (1982). The mnemonic keyword method. *Review of Educational Research, 52,* 61–92.

Purves, D., & Lichtman, J. W. (1985). *Principles of neural development*. Sunderland, MA: Sinauer Associates.

Putnam, H. (1973). Reductionism and the nature of psychology. *Cognition*, 2, 131–146.

Pylyshyn, Z. W. (1984). *Computation and cognition: toward a foundation for cognitive science*. Cambridge, MA: MIT Press

Pylyshyn, Z. W. (1989). Computing in cognitive science. In M. I. Posner (Ed.), *Foundations of cognitive science* (pp. 49–92). Cambridge, MA: MIT Press.

Quartz, S. R., & Sejnowski, T. J. (1997). The neural basis of cognitive development: A constructivist manifesto. *Behavioral and Brain Sciences*, 20, 537–596.

Rakic, P. (1993). Intrinsic and extrinsic determinants of neocortical parcellation: A radial unit model. In M.H. Johnson (Ed.), *Brain maturation and cognition: A reader* (pp. 93–111). Oxford, UK: Blackwell.

Rauscher, F. H., Shaw, G. L., Levine, L. J., Wright, E. L., Dennis, W. R., & Newcomb, R. L. (1997). Music training causes long-term enhancement of preschool children's spatial–temporal reasoning. *Neurological Research*, 19, 2–8.

Raynor, K., & Pollatsek, A. (1989). *The psychology of reading*. Englewood Cliffs, NJ: Prentice-Hall.

Recanzone, G. H., Schreiner, C. E., & Merzenich, M. M. (1993). Plasticity in the frequency representation of primary auditory cortex following discrimination training in adult owl monkeys. *Journal of Neuroscience*, 13, 87–103.

Reichardt, L. F., & Farinas, I. (1997). Neurotrophic factors and their receptors. In W. M. Cowan, T. M. Jessell, & S. L. Zipursky (Eds.), *Molecular and cellular approaches to neural development* (pp. 220–258). New York: Oxford University Press.

Reschly, D. J., & Gresham, F. M. (1989). Current neuropsychological diagnosis of learning problems: A leap of faith. In C. R. Reynolds & E. Fletcher-Janzen (Eds.), *Handbook of clinical child neuropsychology* (pp. 503–519). New York: Plenum Press.

Resnick, L. B., & Omanson, S. F. (1987). Learning to understand arithmetic. In R. Glaser (Ed.), *Advances in instructional psychology* (Vol. 3, pp. 41–95). Hillsdale, NJ: Erlbaum.

Robbins, T. W., & Everitt, B. J. (1995). Arousal systems and attention. In M. S. Gazzaniga (Ed.), *The cognitive neurosciences* (pp. 703–720). Cambridge, MA: MIT Press.

Rothbart, M. K. (1994). Emotional development: Changes in reactivity and self-regulation. In P. Ekman & R. J. Davidson (Eds.), *The nature of emotion* (pp. 369–372). New York: Oxford University Press.

Rumelhart, D. E. (1989). The architecture of mind: A connectionist approach. In M. I. Posner (Ed.), *Foundations of cognitive science* (pp. 133–160). Cambridge, MA: MIT Press.

Sapolsky, R. M. (1999). Glucocorticoids, stress, and their adverse neurological effects: Relevance to aging. *Experimental Gerontology*, 34, 721–732.

Schmidt, L. A. (1999). Frontal brain electrical activity in shyness and sociability. *Psychological Science*, 10, 316–320.

Schmidt, L. A., Fox, N. A., Goldberg, M. C., Smith, C. C., & Schulkin, J. (1999). Effects of acute prednisone administration on memory, attention and emotion in healthy human adults. *Psychoneuroendocrinology*, 24, 461–483.

Schneider, F., Grodd, W., Weiss, U., Klose, U., Mayer, K. R., Nagele, T., & Gur, R. C. (1997). Functional MRI reveals left amygdala activation during emotion. *Psychiatry Research—Neuroimaging*, 76, 75–82.

Scott, S. K., Young, A. W., Calder, A. J., Hellawell, D. J., Aggleton, J. P., & Johnson, M. (1997). Impaired auditory recognition of fear and anger following bilateral amygdala lesions. *Nature*, 385, 254–257.

Searle, J. R. (1992). *The rediscovery of the mind*. Cambridge, MA: MIT Press.

Segal, N. L. (1989). Origins and implications of handedness and relative birth weight for IQ in monozygotic twin pairs. *Neuropsychologia, 27,* 549–561.

Seidenberg, M. S., & McClelland, J. L. (1989). A distributed, developmental model of word recognition and naming. *Psychological Review, 96,* 523–568.

Sejnowski, T. J., & Churchland, P. S. (1989). Brain and cognition. In M. I. Posner (Ed.), *Foundations of cognitive science* (pp. 301–358). Cambridge, MA: MIT Press.

Shaywitz, S. E. (1996). Dyslexia. *Scientific American, 94,* 98–104.

Shaywitz, S. E., Escobar, M. D., Shaywitz, B. A., Fletcher, J. M., & Makuch, R. (1992). Evidence that dyslexia may represent the lower tail of a normal distribution of reading ability. *New England Journal of Medicine, 326,* 144–150.

Shaywitz, S. E., Shaywitz, B., Fletcher, J. M., & Escobar, M. D. (1990). Prevalence of reading disability in boys and girls. *Journal of the American Medical Association, 264,* 998–1005.

Shaywitz, S. E., Shaywitz, B., Pugh, K. R., Fulbright, R. K., Constable, R. T., Mencl, W. E., Shankweiler, D. P., Liberman, A. M., Skudlarksi, P., Fletcher, J. M., Katz, L., Marchione, K. E., Lacadie, C., Gatenby, C., & Gore, J. C. (1998). Functional disruption in the organization of the brain for reading in dyslexia. *Proceedings of the National Academy of Science, 95,* 2636–2641.

Shimamura, A. P. (1995). Memory and frontal lobe function. In M. S. Gazzaniga (Ed.), *The cognitive neurosciences* (pp. 803–813). Cambridge, MA: MIT Press.

Siegler, R. S. (1991a). *Children's thinking* (2nd ed.). Englewood Cliffs, NJ: Prentice-Hall.

Siegler, R. S. (1991b). Strategy choice and strategy discovery. *Learning and Instruction, 1,* 89–102.

Simon, H. A. (1996). *The sciences of the artificial* (3rd ed.). Cambridge, MA: MIT Press.

Smith, E. E., Jonides, J., & Koeppe, R. A. (1996). Dissociating verbal and spatial working memory using PET. *Cerebral Cortex, 6,* 11–20.

Solanto, M. V. (1998). Neuropsychopharmacological mechanisms of stimulant drug action in attention-deficit hyperactivity disorder: A review and integration. *Behavioural Brain Research, 94,* 127–152.

Sprengelmeyer, R., Young, A. W., Calder, A. J., Karnat, A., Lange, H., Homberg, V., Perrett, D. I., & Rowland, D. (1996). Loss of disgust-perception of faces and emotions in Huntington's disease. *Brain, 119,* 1647–1665.

Squire, L. R. (1987). *Memory and brain.* New York: Oxford University Press.

Squire, L. R. (1989). On the course of forgetting in very long term memory. *Journal of Experimental Psychology: Learning, Memory, and Cognition, 15,* 241–245.

Squire, L. R., & Alvarez, P. (1998). Retrograde amnesia and memory consolidation: A neurobiological perspective. In L. R. Squire & S. M. Kosslyn (Eds.), *Findings and current opinion in cognitive neuroscience* (pp. 75–84). Cambridge, MA: MIT Press.

Squire, L. R., & Knowlton, B. J. (1995). Memory, hippocampus, and brain systems. In M. S. Gazzaniga (Ed.), *The cognitive neurosciences* (pp. 825–837). Cambridge MA: MIT Press.

Stanovich, K. E. (1980). Toward an interactive–compensatory model of individual differences in the development of reading fluency. *Reading Research Quarterly, 16,* 32–65.

Stanovich, K. E. (1986). Matthew effects in reading: Some consequences of individual differences in the acquisition of literacy. *Reading Research Quarterly, 21,* 360–407.

Stanovich, K. E. (1988a). The right and wrong places to look for the cognitive locus of reading disability. *Annals of Dyslexia, 38,* 154–177.

Stanovich, K. E. (1988b). Explaining the differences between the dyslexic and the garden-variety poor reader: The phonological-core variable-difference model. *Journal of Learning Disabilities, 21,* 590–604, 612.

Stanovich, K. E. (1998). Cognitive neuroscience and educational psychology: What season is it? *Educational Psychology Review, 10,* 419–426.

Stanovich, K. E., & Siegel, L. S. (1994). Phenotypic performance profile of children with reading disabilities: A regression-based test of the phonological-core variable-difference model. *Journal of Educational Psychology, 86,* 24–53.

Starkman, M. N., Giodani, B., Gebarski, S. S., Berent, S., Schork, M. A.,& Schteingart, D. E. (1999). Decrease in cortisol reverses human hippocampal atrophy following treatment of Cushing's disease. *Biological Psychiatry, 46,* 1595–1602.

Steele, K. M., Bass, K. E., & Crook, M. D. (1999). The mystery of the Mozart effect: Failure to replicate. *Psychological Science, 10,* 366–369.

Steinmetz, H., Herzog, A., Schlaug, G., Huang, Y., & Lanke, R. (1995). Brain (a)symmetry in monozygotic twins. *Cerebral Cortex, 5,* 296–300.

Streissguth, A. P., Barr, H. M., Sampson, P. D., Darby, B. L., & Martin, D. C. (1989). IQ at age 4 in relation to maternal alcohol use and smoking during pregnancy. *Developmental Psychology, 25,* 3–11.

Streissguth, A. P., Sampson, P. D., Barr, H. M., Bookstein, F. L., & Olson, H. C. (1994). The effects of prenatal exposure to alcohol and tobacco: Contributions from the Seattle Longitudinal Prospective Study and implications for public policy. In H. L. Needleman & D. Bellinger (Eds.), *Prenatal exposure to toxicants: Developmental consequences* (pp. 148–183). Baltimore: Johns Hopkins University Press.

Sweller, J., & Cooper, G. A. (1985). The use of examples as a substitute for problem solving in learning algebra. *Cognition and Instruction, 2,* 59–89.

Sylwester, R. (1995). *A celebration of neurons: An educator's guide to the brain.* Alexandria, VA: Association for Supervision and Curriculum Development.

Talairach, J., & Tournoux, P. (1988). *Co-planar stereotaxic atlas of the human brain.* New York: Thieme Medical.

Teasdale, J. D., Howard, R. J., Cox, S. G., Ha, Y., Brammer, M. J., Williams, S. C. R., & Checkley, S. A. (1999). Functional MRI study of the cognitive generation of affect. *American Journal of Psychiatry, 156,* 209–215.

Thompson, R. A. (1991). Emotion regulation and emotional development. *Educational Psychology Review, 3,* 269–307.

Trafford, A. (1999, September 28). Don't blame the womb. *Washington Post (Health),* p. 6.

Tranel, D., Damasio, H., & Damasio, A. R. (1997). A neural basis for the retrieval of conceptual knowledge. *Neuropsychologia, 35,* 1319–1327.

Tulving, E. (1983). *Elements of episodic memory.* New York: Oxford University Press.

Tulving, E., Kapur, S., Markowitsch, H. J., Craik, F. I. M., Habib, R., & Houle, S. (1994). Neuroanatomical correlates of retrieval in episodic memory: Auditory sentence recognition. *Proceedings of the National Academy of Sciences, 91,* 2012–2015.

Tulving, E., & Psotka, J. (1971). Retroactive inhibition in free recall: Inaccessibility of information available in the memory store. *Journal of Experimental Psychology, 87,* 1–8.

van Dijk, T. A., & Kintsch, W. (1983). *Strategies of discourse comprehension.* New York: Academic Press.

Vellutino, F. R., Scanlon, D. M., Sipay, E. R., Small, S. G., Pratt, A., Chen, R., & Denckla, M. B. (1996). Cognitive profiles of difficult-to-remediate and readily remediated poor readers: Early intervention as a vehicle for distinguishing between cognitive and experiential deficits as basic causes of reading disability. *Journal of Educational Psychology, 88,* 601–638.

Vygotsky, L. S. (1978). *Mind in society: The development of higher psychological processes.* Cambridge, MA: Harvard University Press.

Walsh, V., & Rushworth, M. (1999). A primer on magnetic stimulation as a tool for neuropsychology. *Neuropsychologia, 37*, 125–135.

Weaver, C. A., & Kintsch, W. (1991). Expository text. In R. Barr, M. L Kamil, P. Mosenthal, & P. D. Pearson (Eds.), *Handbook of reading research* (Vol. 2, pp. 230–245). New York: Longman.

Weinberger, N. M. (1998). The music in our minds. *Educational Leadership, 56*, 36–40.

Weiner, B. (1985). An attributional theory of achievement motivation and emotion. *Psychological Review, 92*, 548–573.

Weinstein, C. E., & Mayer, R. E. (1986). The teaching of learning strategies. In M. C. Wittrock (Ed.), *Handbook of research on teaching* (3rd ed., pp. 315–327). New York: Macmillan.

Wentzel, K. R. (1997). Student motivation in middle school: The role of perceived pedagogical caring. *Journal of Educational Psychology, 89*, 411–419.

Whittlesea, B. W. A., & Cantwell, A. L. (1987). Enduring influence of the purpose of experiences: Encoding–retrieval interactions in word and pseudoword perception. *Memory and Cognition, 15*, 465–472.

Wigfield, A., & Eccles, J. S. (1992). The development of achievement task values: A theoretical analysis. *Developmental Review, 12*, 265–310.

Winick, M. (1984). Nutrition and brain development. In M. Winick (Ed.), *Nutrition in the 20th century* (pp. 71–86). New York: Wiley.

Wittrock, M. C. (1991). Relations among educational research and neural and cognitive sciences. *Learning and Individual Differences, 3*, 257–263.

Wolfe, P. (1998). Revisiting effective teaching. *Educational Leadership, 56*, 61–64.

Wolfe, P., & Brandt, R. (1998). What do we know from brain research? *Educational Leadership, 56*, 8–13.

Yerkes, R. M., & Dodson, J. D. (1908). The relation of strength of stimulus to rapidity of habit-formation. *Journal of Comparative Neurology and Psychology, 18*, 459–482.

Zakzanis, K. K. (1998). The subcortical dementia of Huntington's disease. *Journal of Clinical and Experimental Neuropsychology, 20*, 565–578.

Index